ACCESS TO MASS TRANSIT FOR BLIND AND VISUALLY IMPAIRED TRAVELERS

ACCESS TO MASS TRANSIT

FOR BLIND AND VISUALLY IMPAIRED TRAVELERS

Edited by
Mark M. Uslan • Alec F. Peck
William R. Wiener • Arlene Stern

American Foundation for the Blind
New York

ACCESS TO MASS TRANSIT
FOR BLIND AND VISUALLY IMPAIRED TRAVELERS
is ©1990 by
American Foundation for the Blind
15 West 16th Street
New York, NY 10011

The American Foundation for the Blind (AFB) is a national nonprofit organization that advocates, develops, and provides programs and services to help blind and visually impaired people achieve independence with dignity in all sectors of society.

Printed in the United States of America

94 93 92 91 90   5 4 3 2 1

Access to Mass Transit for Blind and Visually Impaired Travelers /
    [edited by] Mark M. Uslan . . . [et al.]
        p.   cm.
    Includes bibliographical references.
    ISBN 0-89128-166-5
    1. Blind--United States--Transportation.   2. Blind--Travel--United
States.   3. Local transit--United States.   I. Uslan, Mark M. 1948-
. II. American Foundation for the Blind.
    HV1598.A34   1990
    362.4'183--dc20   89-18332
                                                            CIP

Access to Mass Transit for Blind and Visually Impaired Travelers was edited by Beatrice V. Jacinto, Associate Editor, American Foundation for the Blind (AFB), who also coordinated its production. Its production was supervised by Natalie Hilzen, Managing Editor, AFB.

Photo credits for this publication appear on page 180.

TABLE OF CONTENTS

FOREWORD

ACCESS—whether to information, education, architectural structures, or equal opportunities for employment and social interaction—is a critical issue for blind and visually impaired people. And, like everyone else, people who are blind or visually impaired not only need the chance to take advantage of all these aspects of life, they also need the physical means to get there. Because of the absolutely essential importance of access, the American Foundation for the Blind (AFB) has made it a focus of organizational efforts, and the publication of *Access to Mass Transit for Blind and Visually Impaired Travelers* is a key part.

A couple of years ago the foundation organized an international conference entitled "The Visually Impaired Traveler in Mass Transit: Issues in Orientation and Mobility" expressly to address the vital issues affecting blind and visually impaired travelers who use mass transit. Speakers from the fields of blindness and transportation were joined by consumers to look at the issues, share their experiences, and learn from each other. The different viewpoints and important information presented at the conference have been integrated in this book as part of AFB's efforts to make the environment more accessible to blind and visually impaired people.

In spite of several federal laws providing for increased accessibility, the blind and visually impaired population is still faced with an environment that reflects society's semiconsciousness about the needs of disabled individuals. However, there is growing awareness of these needs and of people's right to independence. As described in the pages of this book, more and more people throughout the world are becoming increasingly concerned about the needs of blind and visually impaired persons and are doing something about that concern.

Because of the variety of perspectives that it presents, *Access to Mass Transit for Blind and Visually Impaired Travelers* is a resource for professionals in the transit industry who are working toward making their systems more accessible, as well as for professionals in the blindness field who are responsible for training blind and visually impaired persons to adapt to the environment. Its materials are also valuable for consumers, who will find its information on different accommodations in various mass transit systems helpful. We at AFB hope that the issues and ideas discussed here will encourage all those who have already begun the work of making society accessible and others who are interested in advocating for changes in transit systems that will make mass transit a daily part of the lives of blind and visually impaired persons.

William F. Gallagher
President and Executive Director
American Foundation for the Blind

PREFACE

IF ONE WERE TO CATALOG the more often used phrases of the eighties, I'm sure "upward mobility" would be near the top of the list. But as much as the expression means for most Americans, it carries a different meaning for those individuals whose physical—as opposed to economic—mobility is limited because of a disability. Disabled Americans, more than anyone else, know that in order to go up the economic ladder, it is necessary to get to the ladder in the first place.

Unfortunately, the world hasn't been a very welcoming place for many disabled Americans. The obstacles faced are different, of course, for each disabled person. But, overall, the everyday world has been designed by and for people for whom a single stair is neither dangerous nor insurmountable and for whom written instructions are always useful.

Will this ever change? Yes, I believe it will. Recent events in the Senate lead me to believe that the 1990s will be the decade of "outward mobility" for disabled Americans. Specifically, my optimism stems from the Senate's passage of the Americans with Disabilities Act (ADA). This bill represents a major advance—it is the culmination of efforts throughout the 1970s and 1980s—to secure civil rights for disabled persons. The legislation says to millions of Americans who are disabled that discrimination against them will no longer be acceptable or allowable—that they will enjoy the same rights and access to participate in society as do all other Americans.

Simply stated, the ADA would ban discrimination on the basis of disability in the areas of jobs, transportation, public services, public accommodations, and telecommunications, both in the public and private sectors. With regard specifically to transportation, the ADA would require transit operators buying new buses to purchase only those units accessible to people with disabilities. Rail systems and over-the-road coaches would also be required to be more accessible. More thought and attention to design would need to be given to how disabled individuals best utilize transportation services. As I write this, consideration of the ADA is pending in the House of Representatives. All indications point to enactment this year, barring unforeseen difficulties.

As American business and society work to make our world more accessible to blind and visually impaired people and others with disabilities, many questions on how best to accomplish this goal will arise. In particular, because it is so crucial an area, there will be many questions about how to make public transportation more accessible. Readily accessible transportation is perhaps the single most important factor in opening up society to blind and visually impaired persons. After all, if disabled people can't get to offices, factories, shopping malls, and restaurants, it doesn't really matter how much more accessible those facilities become.

For these reasons, the publication of *Access to Mass Transit for Blind and Visually Impaired Travelers* couldn't come at a better time. By presenting the views of authors from different fields who themselves present different perspectives on how to make public transportation more accessible to blind and visually impaired individuals, the American Foundation for the Blind performs a valuable and much-needed service. I hope the ideas offered here find a wide readership, particularly among public transportation designers and policymakers. If they do, I'm sure that the "outward mobility" of blind and visually impaired Americans will be greatly enhanced. And that will be good for all Americans.

Alan Cranston
U.S. Senator

Washington, DC
March 1990

ACKNOWLEDGMENTS

THE EDITORS WOULD LIKE TO THANK the people who were responsible for the conference entitled "The Visually Impaired Traveler in Mass Transit: Issues in Orientation and Mobility" held in Washington, DC, in January 1987. The material in this book was based on papers presented at the conference, which was organized by the American Foundation for the Blind (AFB), with the help of the Washington Metropolitan Area Transit Authority (WMATA) and Washington Orientation and Mobility Association (WOMA).

The editors would like to express their special thanks to the following individuals (given here with their affiliations at the time of the conference):

The members of the AFB Conference Planning Committees: Chet Avery, Rehabilitation Services Administration; Pat C. Bucci, Westchester Lighthouse; Anne Corn, University of Texas at Austin; Saul Freedman, Gerald Miller, and Ed Ruch, AFB; James Newcomer, Bucks County Public Schools; Laura Oftedahl, American Council of the Blind; Ralph Weule, Bay Area Rapid Transit; and Martin Yablonski, Guiding Eyes for the Blind.

Carmen Turner, general manager, Karen Pannell, Norris Smith, and other personnel of WMATA who helped in the on-site simulation sessions; Joan Levy Myers, chairperson, and the members of WOMA who helped as learning facilitators in the on-site simulation sessions; and all the participants in the conference.

Beatrice V. Jacinto, associate editor, AFB, who edited the manuscript for this book and coordinated its production, which included extensive photo research and sustained contact with many authors, and whose exemplary professional and personal qualities helped expedite its publication.

The editors would also like to thank all the people and organizations that provided the photographs used in the book, credits for which appear on page 180.

PART I

MASS TRANSIT FOR BLIND AND VISUALLY IMPAIRED PERSONS: VOICES AND PERSPECTIVES

AS BLIND and visually impaired children move away from infancy, they face the challenge of learning to move about independently. When they first confront the issues of crossing busy streets or using mass transit, the challenges they must overcome become greater. A blind person traveling by subway or bus faces a multitude of problems. In no two subway stations are entrances, staircases, fare booths, or platforms in the same place; audio cues on different trains are widely different; rapid rail communication systems are sometimes good but often ineffective or useless. The location of bus stops varies from street to street, and it is difficult to determine bus numbers or routes. Inconsistency is not the exception but the rule in mass transit structures, and soliciting aid from the public demands special skills.

Helping this special population of blind and visually impaired travelers are orientation and mobility (O&M) specialists, who help define travel problems and work with blind and visually impaired clients and their families and mass transit authorities to seek the best and most practical solutions. Since World War II, these professionals have provided training and helped build their clients' confidence to enable blind and visually impaired persons to move freely within their environments. Today, they have become more involved in the complex and demanding area of mass transportation. Certified and trained on either the undergraduate or graduate level, O&M specialists are uniquely equipped to lead their clients to self-assured mobility. Their individual teaching styles may vary, but the goals they have for their clients—independence, self-confidence, and enhanced lifestyle— do not.

The concerns of O&M specialists have come to the attention of a growing body of transit officials, who are putting blind and visually impaired travelers or their advocates on transit system advisory boards. Improvements and changes in both existing systems and newly planned construction are being implemented to meet the needs of blind and visually impaired riders.

The chapters that follow represent different points of view. Blind and visually impaired travelers, O&M specialists, and transit officials speak out about problems and solutions in mass transit for blind and visually impaired persons. Although all these people—along with designers and urban planners— may have different views from where they individually sit, they are working toward the development of techniques, strategies, and facilities to achieve a mutual goal: independent travel for blind and visually impaired people.

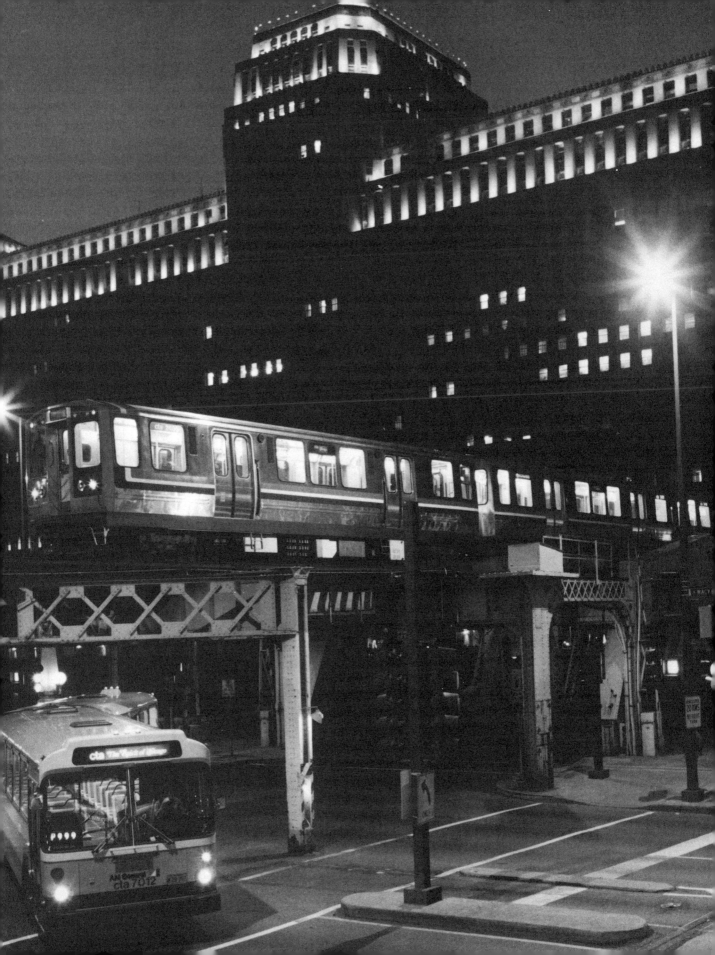

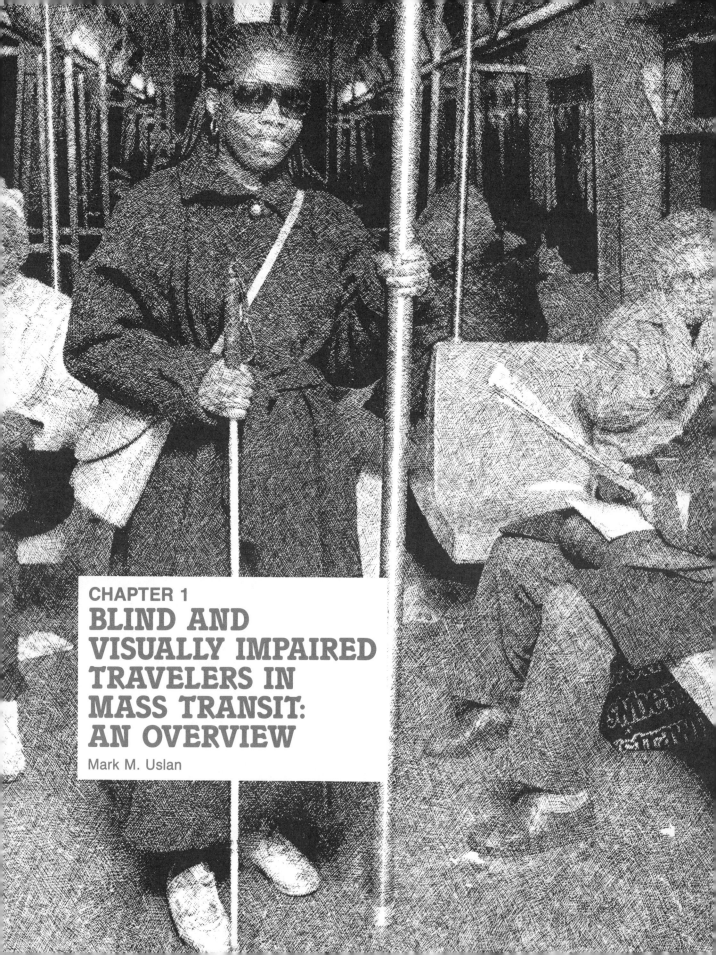

CHAPTER 1
BLIND AND VISUALLY IMPAIRED TRAVELERS IN MASS TRANSIT: AN OVERVIEW

Mark M. Uslan

"But how will you get to work?" is a common question asked by prospective but reluctant employers of blind and visually impaired persons. Independent mobility is often a critical factor in determining whether blind and visually impaired people get jobs and keep them, and maintain a lifestyle of independence and dignity. In response to this question, they should be able to answer with confidence, "Just like anyone else—I'll use the train."

Blind and visually impaired people rely on mass transit to commute to work, shop, meet their friends and family, attend cultural and recreational events—in other words, to do all the things that people with unimpaired vision do. For them to be able to do this, orientation and mobility (O&M) training and an accessible transit system are essential. Furthermore, the cooperation of a wide range of people is involved—the families of blind and visually impaired travelers and their advocates, O&M professionals, rehabilitation counselors, transit personnel, urban planners and architects, manufacturers of transit equipment, and members of the sighted public.

In the early part of this century, disabled people were usually segregated outside the mainstream of society. Dependency and institutionalization were the norm. Blind and visually impaired people who were employed did not commute to their jobs because they worked in settings that provided special residential accommodations (Koestler, 1976; Irwin, 1955).

Over the past 50 years, there has been a growing realization that all disabled people have the right to participate fully in society and to become as independent as they can be. Two federal laws recognizing these rights were enacted in the 1970s. First, the Rehabilitation Act of 1973 forbade discrimination in federal employment, established an Architectural and Transportation Barriers Compliance Board, and, in Section 504, prohibited discrimination against disabled persons in any federally assisted program. Second, P.L. 94-142, the Education for All Handicapped Children Act of 1975, mandated that handicapped children receive a free, appropriate education in the least restrictive environment and thereby embodied the concept of "mainstreaming" children in public schools. In 1989, the Senate passed the Americans with Disabilities Act (ADA), which bans discrimination against disabled persons in the workplace, in transportation facilities, and in public accommodations.

Largely as a result of the major legislation of the last quarter century, today more disabled people than ever lead lives of independence and dignity. Special provisions for the transportation needs of disabled persons can be found in the Urban Mass Transportation Act of 1964, the Architectural Barriers Act of 1968, the National Mass Transportation Act of 1974, and U.S. Department of Transportation regulations implementing Section 504 of the Rehabilitation Act. In addition, the AMTRAK Improvement Act of 1973 authorizes provisions for making intercity rail service accessible, and the Federal-Aid Highways Act of 1973 requires that streets built with federal funds be equipped with curb cuts to provide easy access for those who are in wheelchairs or have other motoric disabilities.

As a result of these changes brought about by legislation, more and more options have become available to blind and visually impaired persons and other disabled populations. Increasing numbers of blind and visually impaired people are migrating to urban areas, where they can move about independently because of extensive mass transit systems. They use buses and subways to go about their daily lives in the mainstream of society. However, more needs to be done to provide all disabled people with the opportunity to be full participants in society. Implementing legislation takes time and money; it may be many years and many millions of dollars before the full impact of the legislation will be felt.

Blind and Visually Impaired Travelers: A Profile

How many people in the United States are blind or visually impaired? Where do they live, and what are their mass transit needs? It has been estimated that as of 1989, 3.5 million people in this country had a severe visual impairment, that is, they could not read ordinary newspaper print (Social Research Department, AFB, 1989, unpublished). For specific administrative purposes, the term "legal blindness" is used to describe a person who has a corrected visual acuity of 20/200 or a visual field of 20 degrees or less. A person with a measured visual acuity of 20/200 can see at 20 feet what persons with normal vision can see at 200 feet. This definition became part of the Aid to the Blind Act of 1935 and, therefore, part of the federal law (Scholl, 1986). Approximately 600,000 persons met the legal definition of blindness in 1987 (Social Research Department, AFB, 1989, unpublished). Legal blindness is a definition that seldom correlates to functional ability, especially in regard to mobility. Many visually impaired people are not legally blind, but they have severe mobility problems under conditions of glare, low contrast, or dim lighting.

It is believed that the legally blind population grew by 12 percent from 1980 to 1990. Today, legally blind persons who are under age 22 represent approximately 8 percent of this population and persons who are 65 and older represent 54 percent. During the period from 1980 to 1990, it is estimated that the 65 and older blind population grew by 17 percent, and the smaller population under age 5 grew by 19 percent (Uslan, 1983).

It has been estimated that 80 percent of the legally blind persons in this country are not totally blind; these individuals can see more than just the presence of light (National Society to Prevent Blindness, 1980). It is also generally believed that there are more blind and visually impaired people who have additional disabilities than those who do not (Kirchner & Peterson, 1988b).

In 1977, 34 percent of all severely visually impaired persons lived in central cities, and another 27 percent lived in either small cities or suburbs of large cities (Kirchner & Peterson, 1988a). The availability of mass transit systems in such areas may be one reason why large numbers of blind and severely visually impaired persons live in or near cities. Although there are no statistics that document why a large proportion of this special population lives in urban areas or how many use mass transit, a well-developed mass transit system must certainly be attractive to blind and visually impaired people who value an independent lifestyle that may or may not include employment.

Blind and visually impaired people experience different degrees of vision loss as a result of their particular visual impairments, and they therefore have widely differing needs. A congenitally blind person is someone who is blind from birth or who became blind at a very early age and therefore needs to learn concepts that would have otherwise been acquired through sight. Being born blind implies a different set of needs than becoming blind later in life does. An adventitiously blind person is someone whose blindness was acquired or caused by an accident. People with adventitious blindness formerly had sight and consequently have visual memory, but they need to master a new set of coping strategies to deal with the world in a nonvisual way safely and effectively. A significant number of blind and visually impaired persons also have disabilities whose presence may complicate their ability to be independently mobile by presenting additional challenges that can be as encompassing as blindness itself. For example, when deafness is added to blindness, the learning of various communication systems such as sign language and finger spelling becomes critically important.

Legal blindness does not imply a particular set of special needs that are present and must be met in every case. Some legally blind people have significant vision and may not need any assistance in using mass transit. Others may only need reassurance and confidence building to be comfortable in dealing with the particular visual and other sensory cues that are available to them. Still others, especially totally blind persons, may have many special needs in the mass transit environment.

The vast majority of totally blind and visually impaired people who need assistive devices for mobility use canes that are specially designed for blind people and for use with certain techniques developed by O&M specialists (Organization for Social and Technical Innovation, 1968). Individuals who choose to use dog guides receive training at one of the specialized schools designed for this purpose.

For those visually impaired people who have usable remaining vision, special optical equipment such as hand-held telescopes, may be helpful when it is necessary to scan the environment for landmarks or signs. These people may never need a cane to travel, or they may need one only infrequently, choosing to use a folding cane that can be conveniently unfolded when needed.

Mass Transit Access

An accessible mass transit system is one that is usable by persons with all types of disabilities. A major problem is that different transit systems present different accessibility problems, and persons with different disabilities require different accommodations. In a few instances, an accommodation for people with one disability may create additional problems for people with another disability; for ex-

ample, curb cuts provide access for persons in wheelchairs but may make it harder for some blind and visually impaired persons to detect where the sidewalk ends and the street begins.

In a handbook on the rights of disabled persons, Charles D. Goldman recounts his experiences while using mass transit exclusively on a trip from Washington, DC, to Brooklyn, New York (Goldman, 1987). The trip entailed riding buses, subways, and an intercity passenger train and included making numerous station changes and using several transit systems of varying ages. Goldman notes that the accessibility of transit systems varies tremendously and that people with disabilities would have encountered diverse problems in the different systems he used on a single trip.

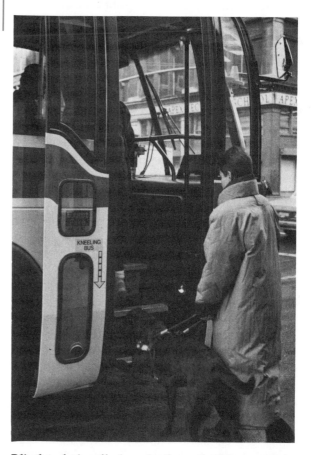

Blind and visually impaired people, like everyone else, use mass transit to go about their daily activities.

In general, making a mass transit system accessible to blind and visually impaired persons seldom requires that structures undergo major redesign to overcome physical barriers, which is often the case with accommodations for persons who use wheelchairs. More often than not, what is required is the clear and appropriate communication of information on a system's layout and its operations, as well as helpful attitudes on the part of transit personnel. Attempting to negotiate a transit system without sufficient information exposes blind and visually impaired persons to a high degree of risk of becoming disoriented and injured.

Many special accommodations that enhance safety and accessibility for blind and visually impaired travelers can also benefit other members of the community. Some examples are schedules and maps in large print for people with low vision or in an appropriate medium for persons who cannot see print; large, high-contrast maps that can be easily read and are prominently displayed in well-lighted, nonglare areas accessible for close examination; and reliable public address systems for the announcement of upcoming stops. Public address systems should be tested and maintained regularly, and announcements should be understandable. Vehicle operators and other personnel having contact with the public need training to be able to recognize when a blind or visually impaired person may need assistance and to be able to respond to those needs effectively. As more is learned about the unique accessibility problems faced by blind and visually impaired travelers using mass transit, new and better ways to make systems accessible will be found.

Orientation and Mobility Training

By themselves, measures to make a mass transit system accessible are not enough to ensure that every blind or visually impaired person will be able to use the system. A person who is blind or visually impaired needs to have the motivation to travel independently and to learn the skills necessary for using the system safely and efficiently. For a few, learning to use mass transit comes naturally, without any type of special instruction; for most, it requires a

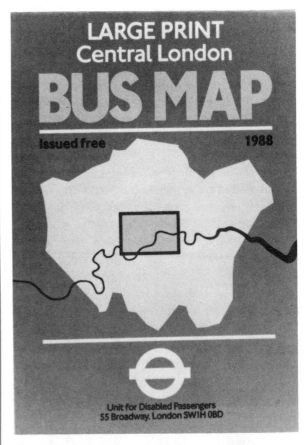

Large-print maps are a special accommodation that contributes to a transit system's accessibility.

significant investment of time and effort, including structured learning experiences.

Without instruction, even the most accessible transit system can be difficult for many blind and visually impaired people to learn to master. Therefore, human service systems need to deliver instructional help through O&M specialists. Certified by the Association for Education and Rehabilitation of the Blind and Visually Impaired (AER), O&M specialists can be found in a variety of settings, including residential rehabilitation centers and schools and itinerant rehabilitation and education programs (American Foundation for the Blind, 1988). Typically, residential rehabilitation centers are administered by an agency of the state, a private nonprofit agency, or the U.S. Department of Veterans Affairs (formerly the Veterans Administration) (VA). Itinerant programs are offered by state or private agencies and public schools.

The responsibility of O&M specialists is to teach blind and visually impaired people how to travel independently in all pedestrian environments, including rapid rail and bus systems. A key aspect of this job is teaching blind and visually impaired people how to use a cane. The systematic use of a cane to travel independently was developed by the forerunners of today's O&M specialists in VA hospitals during and after World War II. From their early work with blinded veterans the touch technique was developed.

In the touch technique, blind and visually impaired people are taught to walk, swinging a cane just above the ground in an arc wide enough to cover the forward path of travel; the cane tip is supposed to touch the ground in synchrony with each footstep, at the far right and left of the path. Special adaptations of the technique assist the cane traveler in two skills important in the mass transit environment, namely, detecting drop-offs and following path edges (Uslan & Schreibman, 1980). All instruction is given on a one-to-one basis and, whenever possible, under real travel conditions, such as in an operating transit system.

From their real-world vantage point, O&M specialists see firsthand the needs of blind and visually impaired travelers, the fears and frustrations of these travelers, the apprehensions of family members, the effect of patronizing public attitudes, and the intricacies of negotiating sophisticated and potentially dangerous travel environments. O&M specialists provide instruction on how to use the cane to probe the environment safely, how to stay oriented when traveling, how to negotiate mazelike environments, and how to obtain and interpret critical travel information from the transit system and from other travelers.

Transit authorities are finding that O&M specialists can help them, too. O&M specialists can train vehicle operators and other personnel to respond to and recognize the needs of blind and visually impaired persons. Training transit personnel to anticipate the needs of blind and visually impaired travelers results in transit operations that run smoothly and with fewer disruptions.

O&M specialists can also help design public education programs to reach blind and visually impaired persons. These programs pay dividends in improved safety records. By convening advisory groups that include blind and visually impaired persons and O&M specialists, transit authorities are finding that they can get useful advice and feedback and, at the same time, generate goodwill.

Partners with Different Perspectives

The intent of this resource book is to foster understanding about blind and visually impaired travelers in mass transit by sharing perspectives, solutions, resources, and strategies. A theme running through the book is the need for partnerships. Blind and visually impaired persons, parents of blind and visually impaired children, O&M specialists, counselors, teachers, transit professionals, urban plan-

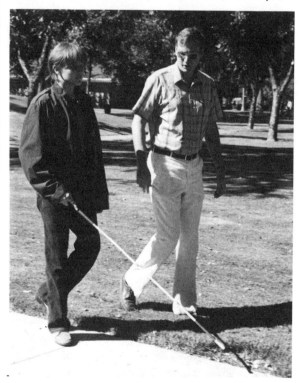

Orientation and mobility instructors are specialists who teach blind and visually impaired people techniques that enable them to travel independently.

ners, architects, designers, and manufacturers are some of the many partners who need to share information and work together if blind and visually impaired people are to travel independently using mass transit.

The perspective of blind and visually impaired travelers provides insights and reveals analyses of transit systems. By relating their firsthand experiences, they provide other mass transit riders with a better appreciation of the frustrations of encountering a myriad of obstacles and the exhilaration of ultimately overcoming those obstacles and traveling safely and independently. The perspective of blind and visually impaired travelers dramatizes the nature of the problems and their solutions.

The perspective of the O&M specialist emphasizes the importance of on-site problem solving. O&M specialists offer many insights from their repeated experiences in teaching and observing

blind and visually impaired travelers in transit systems. Their awareness of many specific training issues needs to be shared.

The transit professional's perspective serves to remind us of the complexities, sophistication, and expense involved in running a modern transit system designed above all to move large numbers of people effectively from place to place. It is not hard to see that a large transit system has its work cut out if it is to achieve its primary objective and that there may always be some problems when attempting to meet everyone's needs all the time.

These three perspectives—from blind and visually impaired travelers, O&M specialists, and transit professionals—provide a wealth of information on how to improve the accessibility of mass transit for blind and visually impaired persons. Taken together, this information provides a blueprint for anyone who wants to help blind and visually im-

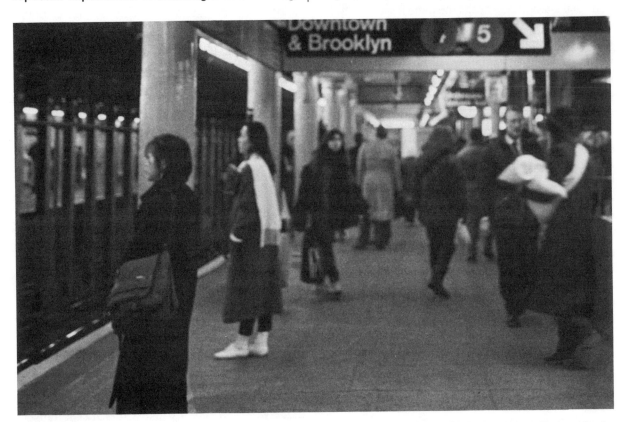

Busy stations with inconsistent structures are some of the challenges that confront blind and visually impaired travelers daily.

paired people achieve the twin goals of freedom through independence and integration into the mainstream of society as safely and as easily as possible.

Gathered from papers presented at a conference entitled "The Visually Impaired Traveler in Mass Transit: Issues in Orientation and Mobility" held in Washington, DC, in January of 1987, the material presented in the chapters that follow shows what has been done, what is being done, and what needs to be done here and in other countries to make mass transit accessible to blind and visually impaired travelers. This handbook addresses blind and visually impaired people and their families, O&M specialists, transit personnel, advocates, and all those working to improve mass transit accessibility for blind and visually impaired travelers.

References

American Foundation for the Blind (AFB). (1988). *Directory of services for blind and visually impaired persons in the United States, 23rd edition.* New York: Author.

Goldman, C. (1987). *Disability rights guide.* Lincoln, NE: Media Publishing.

Irwin, R.B. (1955). *As I saw it.* New York: American Foundation for the Blind.

Kirchner, C., & Peterson, R. (1988a). Data on visual disability from NCHS, 1977. In C. Kirchner (Ed.), *Data on blindness and visual impairment in the U.S.* (2nd ed.). New York: American Foundation for the Blind.

Kirchner, C., & Peterson, R. (1988b). Multiple impairments among noninstitutionalized blind and visually impaired persons. In C. Kirchner (Ed.), *Data on blindness and visual impairment in the U.S.* (2nd ed.). New York: American Foundation for the Blind.

Koestler, F.A. (1976). *The unseen minority: A social history of blindness in the United States.* New York: David McKay.

National Society to Prevent Blindness. (1980). *Vision problems in the U.S.* New York: Author.

Organization for Social and Technical Innovation, Inc. (OSTI). (1968). *Blindness and services to the blind in the United States.* Cambridge, MA: Author.

Scholl, G.T. (1986). What does it mean to be blind? Definitions, terminology, and prevalence. In G.T. Scholl (Ed.), *Foundations of education for blind and visually handicapped children and youth: Theory and practice.* New York: American Foundation for the Blind.

Social Research Department, AFB. (1989). Prevalence estimates of blindness and visual impairment in the United States: Late 1980s. Unpublished data.

Uslan, M.M. (1983). Provision of orientation and mobility in 1990. *Journal of Visual Impairment & Blindness,* **77**(1), 213-215.

Uslan, M.M., & Schreibman, K. (1980). Drop-off detection in the touch technique. *Journal of Visual Impairment & Blindness,* **74**(5), 179-182.

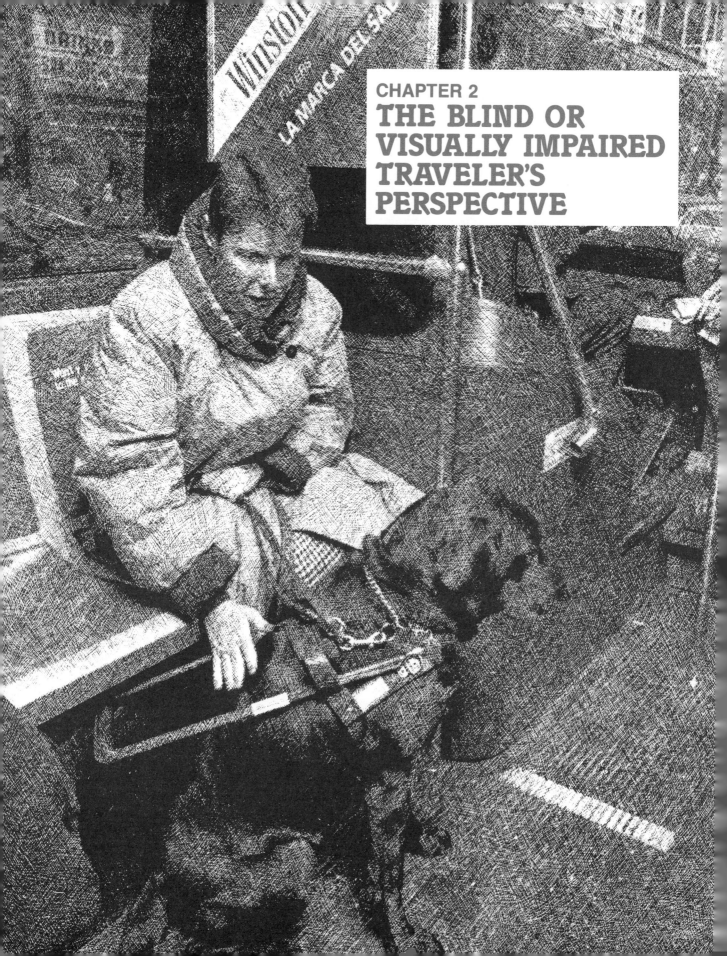

CHAPTER 2
THE BLIND OR VISUALLY IMPAIRED TRAVELER'S PERSPECTIVE

The Challenges of Mass Transit

Anne L. Corn

Blind and visually impaired travelers in mass transit face many challenges negotiating different types of transit systems. In many major cities, consumer panels are organized for the specific purpose of discussing problems encountered by the public in the transit system and recommending solutions. By listening to consumers, transit authorities can learn about challenges that are often created by personnel unaware of people's special needs, exaggerated by physical barriers, or eliminated by problem solving.

At the international conference entitled "The Visually Impaired Traveler in Mass Transit: Issues in Orientation and Mobility" held in Washington, DC, on January 11-12, 1987, five individuals were asked to participate in a consumer panel to discuss some of the problems and challenges encountered by blind and visually impaired people in mass transit travel. Just as consumer panels are convened by transit authorities, this panel was brought together to raise the issues that would be further explored at the conference.

The panel consisted of two totally blind persons, one who travels with a cane and another who travels with a dog guide, and two visually impaired persons, one with peripheral field restrictions and a hearing impairment and the other with low visual acuity with photophobia. A parent of a college student who experienced gradual loss of vision during his high school years was also part of the panel: with training from a mobility instructor, the assistance of his parents, and the use of a cane, the young man has become an independent traveler. The comments, concerns, and recommendations of the members of the panel have been organized in the following pages for the benefit of other consumers, transportation planners and personnel directors, orientation and mobility (O&M) instructors, and others who are interested in the enhancement of independent travel for blind and visually impaired individuals.

Meeting Personal Challenges

Fear and freedom from fear in travel come to different individuals in different ways. Building self-confidence is a major challenge for visually impaired travelers undergoing O&M instruction. For their parents, the challenge is to overcome their anxieties.

I used to walk around my school and my neighborhood just being and feeling totally, wonderfully free. I don't remember being afraid at all. As a young person, I remember beginning to be afraid when I went to a school for the blind in a large city. From that point on, I remember that fear became a part of travel. . . . I chose to travel with a dog guide because I found that it allowed me to move with ease and speed. And from my perspective, right now, as a single woman in New York City, a dog is hard to beat as a travel aid.

My son, Jeffrey, has had retinitis pigmentosa since he was 6 and the disease progressed so rapidly he is now almost totally blind. Even though he had O&M training while he was in high school, he had to begin a very intensive program after his drastic vision loss

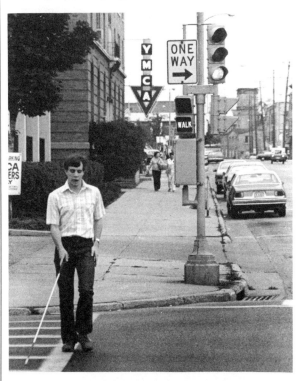

Blind and visually impaired persons who have had training in independent travel become confident in their ability to explore their environment.

in the fall of 1985. This was essential to restore his self-confidence and his ability to function in the outside world.

As our children become teenagers, we need to realize that public transportation is a viable alternative to cars and allows them to go places and do things on their own even though there are risks. As a parent, you're never quite sure whether your child has had sufficient O&M training before you send him or her out on a long trip. You must always display confidence that your child can do it. If you don't, the child very quickly senses your fears and doubts about the situation and will probably resist the effort to learn to travel independently using public transportation. . . .

I remember when I was 17 years old at St. Paul's, now the Carroll Center, when I was handed my first cane. That was a moment of excitement in my life. . . because I was liberated! And that sense of liberation, I think, is commensurate with being 8 years old and getting one's first bicycle or being 16 and getting a license to drive a car. All of a sudden the world was out there!

Success in travel experiences can help individuals gain or regain confidence in their ability to function in an environment primarily designed for sighted persons.

Independent travel using public transportation was a major confidence builder for Jeffrey while he made the painful transition from a visually impaired child to a nearly blind young adult.

I learned from parents that one of the greatest things mobility instruction does is give them information about what their child is capable of doing.

Over Thanksgiving, I was up in a small town in New Hampshire visiting my sister. My family was constantly around me and didn't want me to walk around on my own or walk into town by myself because it was an unfamiliar environment for me. I started feeling very dependent. On the fourth day I developed a severe case of claustrophobia and walked into the town. I didn't have any problems. It was just so important for me to realize that I could do it. I think the same goes for public transportation. One has to rise to the challenges. The more you face them, the more self-confident you become.

Developing desirable approaches and attitudes toward traveling will benefit the individual who is blind or visually impaired. Participants on the panel were asked to rank order desirable personality traits.

I would say assertiveness, coupled with the ability to stay calm and not to take things personally, is very critical. It's important to stay centered and poised . . .and be aggressive, but. . .the gentle kind of assertiveness that allows you to still be in control of the situation. . . . Sometimes you can get into a situation that requires a lot of patience. For example, you get on a subway car, and you're fine. All you're carrying is a purse. A pregnant woman with 16 packages insists on getting up and giving you her seat—and she drops all her packages while she's trying to do it. But she still insists you take her seat. It can really wreck my day and my ability to negotiate safely if I allow myself to feel demeaned, insulted, angry, and embarrassed by such incidents.

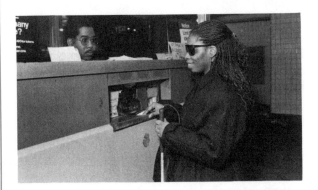

Effective communication skills are essential in soliciting information from transit personnel and the public.

Learning how to solicit information is an important skill that blind and visually impaired travelers need to develop. A visually impaired individual has to determine the best people to ask for accurate directions. He or she must also know how to phrase questions in order to receive appropriate information or confirm prior information.

Ask the proper questions and think how to ask a question. I never just say "Is this on my left or my right?" I always point because I don't want them to have a chance to say what they think left or right is.

Another person you could ask for information is the person you're going to visit. . .people can give you very good directions on how to get to their homes.

. . . When you travel, ask people at the bus stop which bus is coming.

As I talked with other visually impaired people in preparation for this presentation today, one of the things I got was. . . . "Find out as much as you can about the route in advance."

The best person I found to ask was a blind man who grew up in New York City. . . . he could tell me exactly where to stand on a platform so I could get in a specific car and where I would go when I got off in relation to the exit.

Although a cane is not needed by a large segment of the visually impaired population, some individuals will choose to use one, particularly those who have very limited vision under certain environmental conditions. Those who are in the process of gradually losing their vision must determine when a cane is beneficial for mobility and when they are ready to consider it a tool of independence rather than a symbol of vision loss.

I find that when one has one foot in the sighted world and the other in the blind world, this presents other sets of problems. For instance, I don't use a cane even though I should. It'll take some time before I can come to that. In using the transportation system, however, a cane is a good tool to let other people know that you have a vision problem even if you don't need it for mobility. For example, a lot of times while I'm crossing the street in Washington, people assume that I see them when I don't. . . . I know that if I did use a cane and let other people know that I have a problem with my sight, I would probably save myself a lot of aggravation.

Clear, distinct sounds are utilized by travelers as clues to assist in orientation. These represent permanent, though not continuous, sensory input.

You begin to even use the sounds when you're passing by certain train stations when you're on the train. And just the sound of someone going through a turnstile is useful. It can remind you of which station you're at, because you begin to remember on what level the turnstiles can be found.

Effecting Changes in the System

Cooperation and communication between consumers and transit authorities through consumer

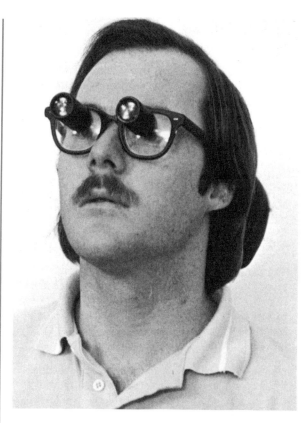

Bioptic telescopes are lenses that are placed on a pair of eyeglasses and used by some visually impaired people to negotiate the environment.

panels can benefit blind and visually impaired travelers. The public can make transit authorities aware of structural problems in the system and how they can be improved. Boards and commissions of transit systems may also benefit from the involvement of O&M instructors, who can give them suggestions on what can be done to make travel easier for blind and visually impaired travelers.

We've done a lot in my city in this area. At my agency we've always had a staff person who is visually impaired on the transit system's advisory committee. One of the problems we had is that our public transportation company tends to run the agendas. About the time they open up the floor for questions or comments, everybody's para-transit vehicle comes, and it's time to go and nobody gets a chance to have any input . . . the agendas are stacked in terms of talking about wheelchair-lift equipped buses and so forth.

Consumers need to be more assertive in terms of getting our issues on agendas.

I think mobility specialists need to take a look at the environment and the transportation systems that are always changing. I think O&M people should find out where the boards and commissions that affect those systems are and make an effort to apply for membership.

Structural Problems

One problem faced by blind and visually impaired travelers are signs that are hard to see. Small signs may be difficult to read as a train is moving into a station.

The big thing that's made a difference for me is a bioptic [telescopic lens placed in a pair of glasses]. I can use the bioptic to read the destination on a bus. Sunglasses are also extremely important for people with albinism because the glare of the sun can be a real problem.

I fell in love with the New York City subway because it has enormous signs that tell you what station you're coming into, and they're close enough together so someone with my kind of vision could have a chance to read them.

Often, no transit personnel are available when someone needs help. The lack of a consistent structure in subway stations also presents problems for blind travelers; O&M instructors may provide helpful input in the construction and adaptation of transit systems. In lieu of a standardization of structure, a well-defined information system is helpful. For example, the availability and standardization of maps offer assistance to visually impaired individuals.

It helps to know when you walk into a subway station where the token booth is. My favorite question when I walk through the turnstile to the first drop-off is: Is that the stairs or is that the tracks? There's no existing kind of information that makes that clear. There's just nothing standard about that from station to station.

I think that maps for visually impaired people are a valuable tool if you want to get around. They need to be done in a standard format. It would help visually impaired persons who go from one city to another to know maps will be available.

. . .this system is very futuristic...instead of people, there are machines. You have to put your money in machines, but it's difficult to determine where they are. There are no paths; just vast open spaces. Give me the Boston MTA system with its dirty claustrophobic arrangements. The paths are clear. You know that if you walk ten steps beyond the turnstiles you're going to fall into a bed. But here the pathways are so wide. . .

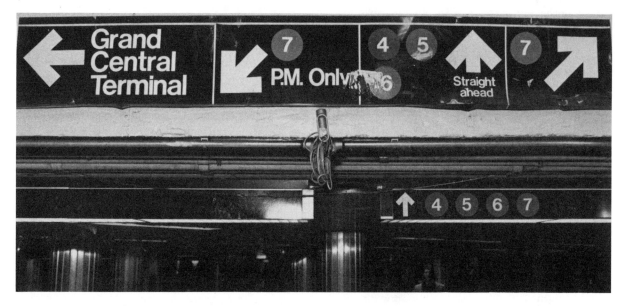

One of the problems faced by visually impaired travelers is confusing and unclear signage.

Lighting is another significant factor that affects travel for visually impaired persons.

I think the Washington Metro is a beautiful system; however, in my personal opinion, the design of the system is so futuristic that it fails to look at decent standards for people with disabilities. The lighting in the system is like twilight. One time I was in the subway and was coming up the stairs from one train to the other line. I saw the train and ran to it because it was standing there. . . . I didn't know that the train was on the other side of the track. So I fell into the track. I think a great deal of it had to do with my having RP [retinitis pigmentosa], but I also think that the lighting was just minimal.

It is important for blind and visually impaired travelers to have a say in structural additions or adaptations because their contributions to decisions regarding such adaptations are indeed helpful.

I understand that on some subways in New York and other places, there are colored places just before you hit the edge of the platform. And I even heard it said that those vary in texture too so you should be able to tell [where you are]. Well, I can't tell if they vary in texture, and I don't think most people can, either.

Challenges Created by Transit Personnel
Common sense and sensitivity are guiding principles that can help transit personnel and the sighted public interact successfully with blind and visually impaired travelers. Problems associated with poor personnel-consumer interactions should be reported in order to correct the situation and to alert transit system personnel to possible recurring problems.

Last summer Jeffrey asked a bus driver to advise him when his particular stop came. The driver mumbled some kind of excuse and refused to help him. He had to ask another passenger for help. My husband and I were outraged at this, and we called the bus company the next day and reported the incident. The following day Jeffrey received an apology from the bus driver. And after that the driver helped him find his point of destination for the rest of the summer.

If bus drivers would just speak, you can find out what you need to know. While I was waiting to get on the bus and I was the first one in line, the door opened and I said, "Is anybody coming out?" Nobody said

a word to me. I got on the bus, and my dog stopped because I couldn't move. The reason I couldn't move was that there was a bunch of people there. Then the driver said to those people, "Go on out of the back!" If the driver will talk to you, no matter what he says, we'll get it together. Talk to me. Don't talk to everybody else about me.

I find that bus drivers really don't know about all disabilities, because sometimes they shout, thinking that blindness is actually deafness. Or they speak very slowly and meticulously. This comes from thinking that blindness is actually mental retardation. Or they drag you, [as if they think] you're in a wheelchair, or that you need to be carried. Bus drivers should be informed that all disabilities aren't the same. . . .

Then there's the problem of when you get on the bus and you ask the driver to tell you to get off at the stop you want, and he forgets to tell you. There are a couple of solutions to that. One is knowing as much as you possibly can about the entire route that the bus is going to take. Know the landmarks. Know how much time it's going to take you to get there approximately. So that just about the time you get there, you can remind the driver to tell you to get off at the stop you want. I've also found that asking other people on the bus can be much more reliable than asking the bus driver.

Solutions
Experiences in traveling with vision-reduction goggles may benefit transit personnel in their understanding of the problems and challenges that confront blind and visually impaired travelers.

I guess as a community service for our bus drivers, we owe it to them and their supervisors to let them feel how visually impaired people feel and give them a little bit of training in how to deal with people. I think a lot of it is not that they don't know how to care. . . . A lot of them are just frightened and don't know how to deal with certain situations. However, if they're presented with a situation and have in-service training for a day on how to deal with all types of disabilities, I think that would help them greatly. They would overcome their fears and be able to deal with things in a positive way.

Proper use of communication devices in transit systems is essential.

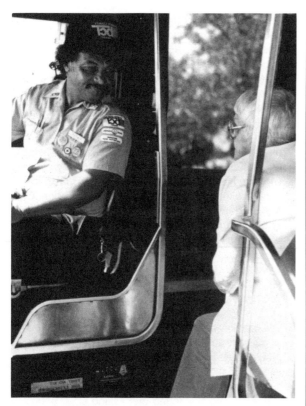

Bus personnel who understand the problems and challenges that confront blind and visually impaired travelers are better able to be of assistance to them.

The old joke about the subways is this: The train starts to go. And the guy says, "Next stop is. . . ." You can't make out a thing. Then he says, "Watch the closing doors." You get that, but you never know what street you just passed. Now I think this has begun to change. I don't know whether they've improved the mikes or they've simply done some commonsense things. For example, train personnel can be trained how to use a microphone [and learn] such things as how far away or close to a mike to be when trying to get a point across. Teach them not to make critical announcements when the train is at its loudest—to wait for a quiet moment. We're even reaching a point now when some of the conductors have the grace and intelligence to say, "Now arriving across the platform, the number two express."

At the same time, blind and visually impaired travelers should acknowledge those persons and practices that benefit them. This rewards a job well done. Also, the practice can be publicized, and other personnel may adopt similar behaviors.

One of the most terrific accommodations that I ever came upon in the subways was done by one particular guy in the token booth with a lot of common sense. When he would see me coming and getting close to his booth, he would turn on his little microphone and just slightly tap on it. It wasn't even that loud. It was just like a little beacon. It was such a pleasure.

I've been delinquent about writing a letter to the MTA [Metropolitan Transit Authority] to congratulate him and to suggest that kind of an idea. . . is one of the most helpful kinds of things.

I would also like to make a suggestion that there be an award program set up by some of the consumer groups and public transportation companies that really focuses on awarding the drivers who are good. We have a driver in Philadelphia on the C bus of Broad Street who is just wonderful. He says good morning to everybody, and he announces every street whether there's a blind person on the bus or not. He always has something pleasant to say as people are getting off. People like him deserve recognition. Perhaps if we award people like him, other people will be a little bit more pleasant, too.

Personnel knowledgeable about the transit problems of blind and visually impaired individuals and, possibly, certified O&M instructors can be hired by transit systems and rehabilitation agencies to act as consultants, or privately hired on a short-term basis by individuals.

If a blind person doesn't necessarily want to get involved with rehab or with the services of an agency, he [or she] could call an O&M person and say, "Hey, here's my problem. I want to get from here to there—could you come out and help me?" without having to deal with all the enrollment paperwork and get involved with the rehab agency. This would be a quick and easy way of getting a guy like me to take some time to know where the subway system is here in Washington.

Excerpts from this consumer panel discussion have been presented here as a beginning to an ongoing dialogue that should continue among blind and visually impaired travelers, transit personnel, and professionals in the field of blindness and visual impairment.

Getting Around in a Major Metropolis: The Experiences of Guide Dog Users in Mass Transit

Edwin Eames
Toni Gardiner Eames

The negative aspects of city life in the United States have often been discussed in literature and the media. For a particular segment of the population, however, cities offer amenities that far outweigh their disadvantages. Blind people are part of this group. For them, the availability of mass transportation is a basic amenity not found in suburban areas. Therefore, it is likely that the major segment of the blind population in the United States lives in urban areas. Unable to drive and desiring independence in travel, they avail themselves of existing transportation facilities.

There are three major public transportation systems available in New York City: buses, subways, and commuter trains. For a blind traveler using a guide dog, particular problems arise in negotiating transportation systems. Our focus here will include some of the problems faced by blind guide dog users in the New York City metropolitan area.

The Public

Although the physical attributes of public transportation in any area are a primary factor in our ability to move around independently, the most important element in a transit system from a blind person's perspective is the public. Sighted people tell us whether the E train or the F train is approaching, where the bus stop is located, or where to find Gate 15 in the railroad station.

A lack of physical uniformity within the system, combined with unreliable communications equipment, makes us more dependent upon the public, which is not always ideal. Sometimes we get several different answers when we ask "What train is this?" Or, while someone is checking, the doors of the train close, and we are left standing on the platform. At other times, in enlisting the aid of a passerby to locate a particular bus stop, we are directed to the nearest one. We wait, a bus pulls up, and the driver informs us that we are waiting at the wrong bus stop. Seeking out another passerby and going through the process all over again takes more time and effort.

When there are no ticket agents in a commuter railroad station, we have to rely on passengers for information on train schedules. Often, other passengers are not reliable. Problems are caused by many factors. Being blind, we are largely dependent on others for such help, but people are frequently in a hurry, and giving directions takes time. Sometimes they do not have the needed information but feel that they should provide it nonetheless, and sometimes they just do not listen carefully to the question. We also come across people who do not speak English or those who do not want to take time to respond. This can be very frustrating.

People can also become oversolicitous and intrusive. This behavior takes a number of forms, but the most common one is grabbing someone who is blind by the elbow and propelling him or her toward the requested destination. When the blind person is getting off a train or approaching a staircase, this unanticipated and unwanted hands-on help can cause disorientation, discomfort, and even injury.

Nonuniform Structures

Blind people's dependency on others is intensified by the lack of uniformity in all systems of mass transportation in most metropolitan areas. Buses sometimes stop at the far corner, sometimes in the middle of the block, and sometimes at the near corner. In addition, buses sometimes stop on odd blocks, at other times on even blocks. There are shelters at some stops but not at others.

The subway system is similarly inconsistent. Some subway stations are entered through staircases located alongside the curb, others by going through a building to the staircase. Stations may be located in the middle of a block or at the end of a block. Token booths, turnstiles, and entrance or exit

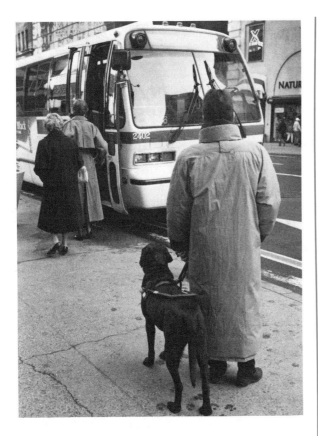

The inconsistent location of bus stops can be a cause of confusion for blind travelers.

gates are located in different places in different stations. In some stations, trains come in at the entrance level; in other stations, one must descend several flights of stairs to get to the platform where the trains arrive; and in still other stations, one has to go up to an elevated structure in order to reach the platform. The types of platforms themselves vary. Similar problems are confronted by blind and visually impaired persons wanting to use the railroad system. Locations and layouts of commuter stations are rarely consistent.

Communication Problems

Blind commuters need clear and concise oral information. Bus drivers should consistently announce stops, and public address systems on subways and commuter trains should transmit intelligible messages at all times. When there is a failure to communicate, we sometimes miss a train, get on the wrong train, or, on rare occasions, get off at the wrong station. Such situations are distressing.

The Bus System

Short bus trips can also present numerous problems. These range from finding the initial location of the bus stop to getting on the correct bus to getting off at the desired final destination.

City Buses

In spite of the lack of consistency in bus stop locations, finding a bus stop can be managed with the help of somebody who can see. It can also be done by deliberately familiarizing oneself with the location and using the stop on a regular basis. Standing within the bus shelter, in cases where one exists, is extremely important because drivers will rarely stop outside the shelter area. Another difficulty is finding the end of the waiting line. If people do not direct us correctly, we may end up breaching the line, which can cause ill will. When buses do not pull up alongside the curb, we must walk off the curb and into possible danger. When more than one bus route uses the same stop, the procedure becomes even more dangerous. A blind traveler must step off the curb, approach the bus, and ask the bus driver which bus it is. Of course, if there are people around, they may provide this information.

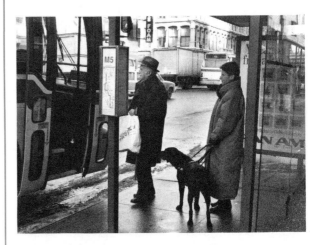

The presence of bus shelters on the street makes it easier for blind travelers to locate bus stops.

After boarding the bus, a whole new set of potentially frustrating situations exists. Finding the fare box may not be easy, because these boxes are not in the same place in all buses. In addition, there is no space under the seats that are reserved for disabled riders on the bus, and it is difficult to protect one's guide dog. Other passengers who board the bus may not see the dog sitting between our knees and may accidentally step on the dog's paws or hit the dog with shopping bags, pocketbooks, or briefcases. If we sit further back in the bus, the dog sits under the seat and is better protected. However, the bus driver is much more likely to forget to tell us when we reach our stop if we are not in his or her immediate vicinity. If we choose to exit the bus from the back door, we have to be extremely careful because the driver might have pulled alongside an obstacle, such as a tree or a pole. Obviously, it is the job of our dogs to avoid such obstacles, but on coming down the two or three steps at the rear door of a bus, this may prove troublesome. Also, the driver may not be able to stop the bus directly alongside the curb, causing a difficult step-down or requiring us to walk several feet to the safety of the curb.

Express and Commuter Buses
Express buses come into the central part of the city from outlying boroughs and suburban areas; fares for these buses are much higher than those for city buses. Placing the fare in the box is a challenge. Almost all these buses require exact change, and when bills are placed in the fare box, they must be placed right side up and centered. Even for the most dexterous blind person who carefully separates his or her bills, there is no way of knowing which side of the bill is right side up. Drivers do not assume responsibility for putting the bills in correctly.

Commuter buses present their share of problems to blind travelers. In an enormous bus terminal like the Port Authority Bus Terminal in New York City, locating the correct ticket window and, subsequently, the correct bus gate can be a frustrating experience. The structure of the new section of the Port Authority Bus Terminal is based upon a cluster principle and is primarily set up for visual identification.

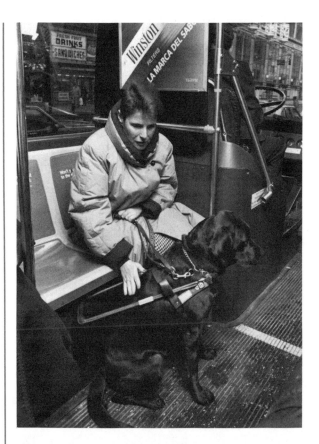

One problem faced by guide dog users on city buses is that usually no space is provided for a dog under the seats reserved for disabled riders.

Getting from the first to the third level of the building by stairs or escalators requires a break in direction and a reorientation because staircases and escalators do not follow a straight-line pattern. This was probably designed to provide some traffic breaks, but for a blind commuter, it creates a nightmare. When we reach the second level, we must find the stairs or escalator to level three, which can be difficult and confusing.

If working one's way through the Port Authority Bus Terminal is difficult, returning to it is as much of a problem. In many outlying areas, particularly in New Jersey, one has to flag down a bus when returning to the city. Unless we are standing in exactly the right place and waving our hand as the bus approaches, there is a strong possibility that the driver will not see us and will pass the stop by.

The Subway System

Using the subway system requires ingenuity and persistence. Even getting into the system presents a formidable challenge.

Paying the Fare

Disabled and visually impaired mass transit riders are only charged half fare. In bus travel, the half-fare discount is easy to handle. One simply puts 55 cents instead of a dollar in the coin box. In subway travel, however, the procedure is much more complicated. The New York system requires the purchase of a token at full price and the receipt of a free return ticket, or the presentation of a previously obtained return ticket at the token booth. At regularly used stations, guide dogs quickly learn to find the booth. But whenever we use a new station or use a station infrequently, finding the token booth can be a trying experience.

If we have a token, we enter the station through a turnstile, but if we present a return ticket, we enter the station through a gate. There are, however, different types of turnstiles and a variety of gates. It is difficult to get a dog, much less ourselves, to sort out the variations on this theme of getting to the train. Subway booth attendants are not trained to direct blind people to the correct entry point. It is at this point that members of the public try to be helpful. As we tell our dogs to find the gate or the turnstile, a passenger is likely to grab us by the arm or pull on the dog's harness handle in an attempt to direct us to the correct entrance. This presumed help interferes with our ability to function. It is rare to find someone who will take the time or who knows how to offer assistance that will enable us to remain in control of the situation.

Locating Platforms

After successfully tackling the challenge of the turnstile or gate, the next chore is to locate the desired

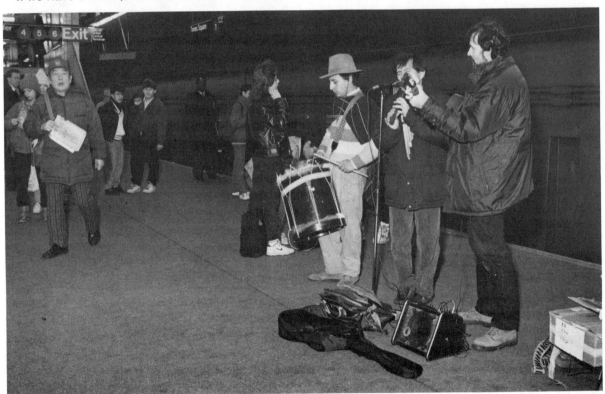

Blind travelers depend on sound localization to help them negotiate train platforms. The presence of additional sources of noise, such as street musicians, makes this difficult.

platform. The platform may be directly in front of the turnstile, but more frequently it is above or below the turnstile entry level. There may be a variety of staircases or escalators leading to various track levels and to trains going in different directions. At one station, northbound and southbound local and express trains use track levels one and three, while eastbound and westbound trains use track level two. The ubiquity of subway street entertainers at this station creates still more confusion. The amplification of their voices and musical instruments reverberates and interferes with one's ability to hear. What lends the situation particular importance is that the station is located near a well-known agency for blind and visually impaired clients who use the station.

Getting to a platform at all can be a problem. Escalators in many subway stations are either the only choice for movement or are more readily accessible or more convenient than the staircases. Most guide dogs, however, are not trained to use escalators. Thus, one faces the inconvenience of trying to locate staircases.

Finding the Right Train

In addition to arriving at the right platform, entering the right train is the next hurdle confronting a blind traveler. Subway platforms are found either on a single-track or a double-track layout, and it is difficult to distinguish one from the other. Most blind people feel safer on a single-track platform, especially if they have to walk along the platform for any distance. The sounds of incoming and outgoing trains may help in orientation, but when they are combined with loud or incomprehensible public announcements and street music as well, the potentially disorienting impact on a blind traveler is often exacerbated.

Listening to Announcements

In our discussions with other blind travelers, the most frequently cited complaint is that already existing communications equipment is not utilized. Every train and most stations have public address systems. Sometimes station announcements are made identifying a train, and at other times iden-

tification announcements can be heard from the train itself. Often, in our experience, no announcements are made at all, or if announcements are made, they are incomprehensible.

After taping and doing a frequency check on train announcements over a 3 month period, we found these results: no announcements were made on one third of the trains; garbled announcements due to poor announcing techniques or faulty equipment were made on an additional one third; and readily understandable and informative announcements were made on another third. When we travel on familiar routes, a lack of information is merely annoying. When we travel on unfamiliar routes, however, a lack of information causes extreme tension. This problem could be readily solved by training employees and maintaining equipment.

The lack of an effective communication system is compounded when two or more trains with different routes and different destinations share the same track. Then we become dependent on sighted passengers to identify oncoming trains. Usually, correct information is obtained, but being dependent on others sometimes leads to our taking the wrong train or missing the train completely. Decisions about boarding a train must be made quickly because the doors remain open for less than one minute.

Getting Off the Train

When leaving the train, blind travelers are faced with many of the same situations they encountered in entering it. These include negotiating a way through half-open doors, around passengers who stand in the open doorway, and among crowds of people who are attempting to enter the train. When exiting at an unfamiliar station, one cannot predict on which side of the train the doors will open; whether the stop will have a single- or double-track platform; where to transfer to the next train, if necessary; whether the exit to the street is on the platform level or up- or downstairs; and which type of turnstile or gate one will have to use to exit. One particularly unwelcome type of gate is the barred revolving gate. In order to negotiate this safely with a guide dog, one must go slowly to make sure that the dog is not caught. Impatient passengers, in their attempt to assist, may push the gate faster than is comfortable for someone with a dog, which can result in an injury.

We often fantasize about a subway system in which station stops and train destinations are announced clearly; the trains are relatively quiet and pull up in a spot convenient to where we are standing; both doors open and we can enter the train without having to push other passengers aside; and we can sit in a relatively clean area. Reality, however, has taught us, or forced us, to deal with trains that stop yards down the platform from where we are standing; doors that do not open at all or open only halfway; and people who block the open door so that our dogs cannot guide us in. Finally, we have to live with having our dogs sit in debris. These problems are not unique to blind passengers, but their impact on us is great.

The Commuter Life

Commuter trains create some unique problems for blind and visually impaired passengers in addition to those problems that we experience in other mass transit systems. When we are traveling out of the city from one of the major railroad terminals, we have to negotiate large, nonstandardized, noisy, and crowded depots. We often need sighted assistance in locating ticket booths, information booths, and track gates, as well as the train itself, since usually two or more trains depart from either side of a platform. Although boarding these trains is not as frantic a procedure as boarding a subway train, the noise and confusion in these stations can be disorienting. When we try to obtain information, the surrounding noise can drown out verbal assistance. After entering the correct train, we must find a seat under which our dogs can lie comfortably and cleanly. And, as in the subways, we often have to strain to hear announcements that are unintelligible.

On leaving the train, we also face a host of problems. Train doors may open only halfway or may not open at all. By the time we get near them, those doors may be in the process of closing, and we miss our stop. More disturbing and far more dangerous

is the situation sometimes seen with diesel trains, in which doors may open when the train has come to a stop but is not at a platform. We may not be aware that the train has stopped for a traffic signal and has not yet arrived at the station. An attempt to disembark at this point would be dangerous.

An additional problem exists on the railroad because of the wide gap between the train and the platform. We have no way of predicting in an unfamiliar station just how wide that gap is, and many passengers have been injured by not taking a large enough stride when getting off the train. The problem is made worse when sighted passengers, attempting to assist, grab us and throw us off balance. Some blind passengers have slipped between the train and the platform when getting off trains, and, in at least one case, a guide dog fell under a train. Train personnel are not always available to help when problems arise.

After exiting the train in an unfamiliar suburban station, a blind or visually impaired passenger may not know whether it is a single-track or a double-track platform. As in the subway, there is no standard platform configuration. Stairs or escalators may have to be found. If a blind passenger is not being met at the station, a telephone or taxi may have to be located. Sighted assistance is almost always necessary because telephones and taxis are never in a set place. There is also the occasional need to walk in front of a stationary train in order to leave the station. Railroad gates provide sighted passengers with visual cues that are not readily accessible to a blind passenger.

In the subway system, sighted assistance is almost always immediately available, but small suburban railroad stations may be deserted. Frequently, ticket offices are closed except during commuter rush hours, and signs are posted containing information about train times and tracks. Obviously, these visual cues are useless to blind and visually impaired people. A blind or visually impaired passenger may feel isolated and vulnerable when a train pulls in far down the platform and, before he or she can reach an open door, the door signal has rung, the doors have closed, and the train has pulled out of the station. One of the authors is a regular commuter on the Long Island Railroad system and, through her own experience, knows that on occasion, eastbound trains come in on westbound tracks, and vice versa, and that passengers, both blind and sighted, are confused when they are not told in what direction the train is traveling.

Problems and Solutions

Blind passengers using the transportation systems in a major metropolis like New York City face a variety of difficulties that are not shared by sighted travelers. Most of these difficulties result from the inability to read visual cues. We are dependent on other sorts of cues, primarily auditory, and, most important, on information received either from the public or from the mass transit system itself. Both these sources can be unreliable and communicating with them is complicated by disorienting noise. Lack of uniformity within the transit system is the basis for many of the difficulties encountered, and buses, subways, and trains all present their own sets of problems to blind and visually impaired travelers.

What can be done to alleviate these frustrating conditions? No one can expect to have any mass transit system rebuilt to his or her specifications. There do seem to be some immediate remedies, however. One major change would entail making the existing communication systems more relevant to the needs of both blind and sighted passengers. Public address systems in stations and communication systems on trains and subways should present information clearly and concisely.

Personnel such as token booth attendants, bus drivers, subway and train conductors, and transit security forces should be trained to increase their awareness of the special requirements of blind persons and other disabled passengers. Techniques to aid blind and visually impaired people need to stress verbal rather than visual information. Personnel should be taught to offer assistance, if it is needed, and not to grab a blind person or touch a working guide dog. This kind of orientation could be incorporated into already existing training programs, with the vital goal of sensitizing the employees of mass transit systems to the needs of special passengers.

The New York City transit system is one of the most comprehensive in the country, allowing travelers to reach widely distant points. Guide dog users—and, of course, long cane users as well—want to get to those points, too, and can work with transit authorities to lessen the hazards, discomfort, and frustrations now inherent in the system. Training, improved communications, and increased uniformity throughout the system would greatly enhance our ability to utilize the system to the fullest.

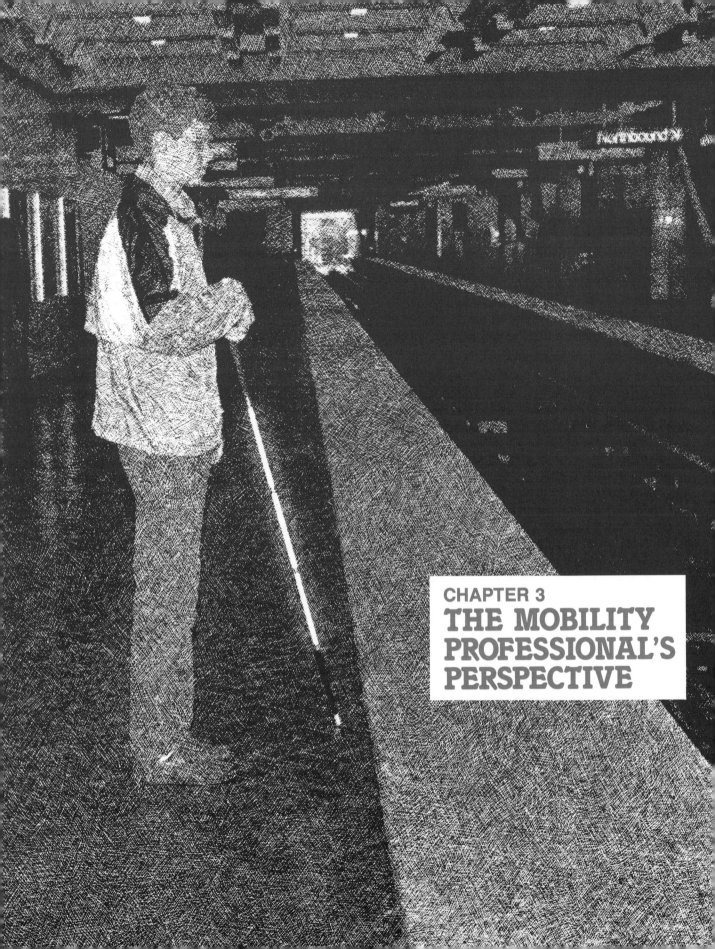

CHAPTER 3
THE MOBILITY PROFESSIONAL'S PERSPECTIVE

Training for Travel in Rapid Rail

William R. Wiener

Orientation and mobility (O&M) specialists are in the front line of teaching and training blind and visually impaired individuals to move safely and efficiently in their environment. Although proud of their clients' achievements, these professionals recognize the problems inherent in the use of mass transit systems —particularly rapid rail—for the constituency they serve. They are an ideal source of information about safe travel for blind and visually impaired travelers.

There are successful strategies and solutions for overcoming the difficulties and dangers of mass transportation. It is incumbent on O&M professionals to work for and achieve an expansion of the O&M curriculum in order to increase their clients' potential for independent travel.

Blind and visually impaired people have been successful in traveling in complex and changing environments. Skilled travelers have learned to analyze and recognize regular features of their surroundings and anticipate irregularities. The more predictable the environment, the easier it is to maintain orientation. The more concrete the landmarks, the easier it becomes to locate and utilize them.

Systems of public transportation are no exception to these rules. To the extent that the systems are predictable, they become easy to negotiate. For example, bus systems that have stops with similar physical layouts have a dimension of familiarity that makes their use much easier. Close proximity of the stops to heavily traveled sidewalks makes them an integral part of the environment. The more the stops become part of that everyday environment, the easier it becomes to predict their location and gain access to them.

Rapid rail travel poses a particular set of problems and a new set of rules for travelers to master. The rapid rail system is often in an isolated environment that is separate and distinct from commonly traveled streets and intersections. Systems are engineered to allow the most efficient movement of large numbers of people in the least amount of time. Unfortunately, the attributes that make a system efficient at moving people do not necessarily make it accessible or easily usable by people with visual disabilities. Often, transit systems are built so as to be understood through visual interpretation, and therefore, information for orientation and for safety may not be available to a blind or visually impaired traveler.

Rapid rail systems create a special below- or above-ground environment that is difficult to interpret. Transit systems often consist of large expansive areas with few tactile landmarks and important conveyances that are inconsistently placed. Signs are displayed for fully sighted individuals and without much thought to the needs of blind and visually impaired people. The very design of typical platforms makes them hazardous to negotiate. There often is no standardization between various stations in a system or between different systems. This leaves passengers to face an unpredictable environment with inadequate information.

General problems common to most systems make travel difficult for blind and visually impaired people. These need to be understood so that techniques for travel can be developed to minimize dangers and maximize the information available.

Defining the Problems

A number of problems are encountered in travel, starting from the beginning when a blind or visually

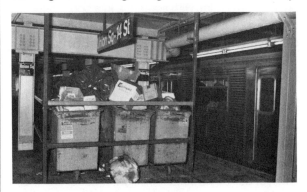

Cluttered platforms are hazardous for travelers who have to walk near the edge of the platform to move from one point to another.

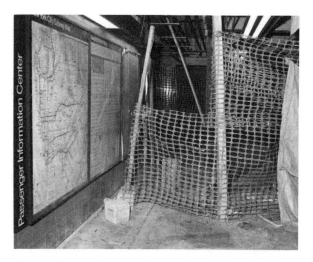

Passenger Information Center

A familiar station may be rendered inaccessible as well as dangerous by unexpected obstacles.

impaired traveler wishes to gain access to a station. Inconsistent signs, or signs that are not in braille or are hard to read or, lack of usable physical landmarks may make it hard to identify stations and locate entrances.

Locating and negotiating public conveyances present the next challenge. It may be difficult to use an escalator in a rush of people. Stairs may be wet and slippery or cluttered with debris. Also, the first stair edge may not be marked with high-contrast warning strips. Handrails may be difficult to locate or may not stretch along the entire length of the stairs.

Travel within the station involves other difficulties. Entrances may be restricted by a fare barrier or ticket booth. Conversing with someone in a booth may be difficult when small openings in the booth impair effective vocal communication. Often, visual information is needed to use farecard machines. Entrances or turnstiles are not located in standard places, and no tactile clues may be available. Narrow turnstiles are difficult for dog guide users to negotiate, and it is often not possible to distinguish between entry and exit turnstiles. It may also be difficult to insert farecards properly or to distinguish token or coin slots because of low contrast and lack of textural differences.

Once through the entrance, a traveler may have trouble locating the correct platform, train, travel direction, and waiting point. Signs may be too high or difficult to read or inconsistently placed. Large-print or tactile maps are generally not available.

Other problems also present themselves as a blind or visually impaired traveler attempts to avoid platform difficulties and hazards. There are often no edge markings or only badly painted lines near the drop-off of the platform. Tactile warning strips, when present, are often worn down. In addition, pavement in bad repair may give misleading clues. Double-track platforms that are cluttered with platform furniture, poles, magazine racks, and other obstacles on the travel path may force a traveler who is trying to walk parallel to the drop-offs to change direction and walk dangerously close to a drop-off.

On the platform, the major task is to identify the correct train and locate the train's entry points. Often, trains are not announced, and there is insufficient signage. Some trains may actually sit silently without a blind or visually impaired person's being aware that they are there. Open spaces between cars can be mistaken for doors and pose potential dangers. In some systems, the gap between the platform and the train may be large enough to catch a passenger's heel, causing a fall. Doors may be unmonitored and may close too quickly.

Once in the train, it may be difficult to determine when the train has reached the desired destination.

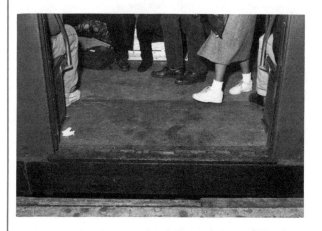

Faded platform-edge markings and large gaps between the train and the platform contribute to the difficulties faced by blind and visually impaired travelers.

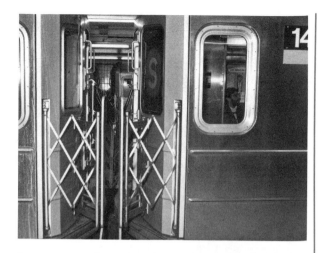

Open spaces between the cars on a train can be dangerous when they are mistaken for entrances to the cars. Safety gates have been installed in some trains to solve this problem.

Usually, stops are announced, but if these announcements are unintelligible, conductors may not be around to provide information. When the train comes to a station, there is frequently no indication of the side of the car on which the doors will open. There also may not be sufficient time to exit before the doors close.

Exiting from a complex station poses additional difficulties. Some platforms are constructed in a way that makes it difficult to locate stairs and escalators, and one may wander to the end of the platform, where a drop-off may exist. Negotiating floor-to-ceiling turnstiles can be hazardous, particularly for a dog guide; in contrast, one may sometimes have to deal with wide-open areas that have few physical boundaries. When walls do exist, they may be constructed of bars rather than built as solid, unbroken expanses and therefore may distort sound location and impair orientation. Some stations contain alleys that lead nowhere. In some systems, the value of a farecard may have to be increased before one can exit. This procedure requires locating special farecard machines and then returning to the turnstile. A blind or visually impaired traveler must learn to anticipate all these problems and use appropriate techniques and strategies to reach his or her destination.

Applying Solutions

O&M specialists have varying degrees of experience with travel in the rapid rail environment. During the latter part of 1986, an informal survey was conducted at Western Michigan University to find out how instructors in various universities that offer O&M training were prepared to teach blind and visually impaired people to travel in rapid rail systems. Thirteen universities were contacted, and ten responses were received. Staff at the universities were asked to explain if rapid rail travel was covered in their respective curricula; how it was presented to the students if it was covered; what practical experiences students received; and what particular solutions to problems seemed most promising. The survey results indicate that instruction in this area is inconsistent. Programs that are in close proximity to rapid rail systems often are able to provide their students with direct experience. Others, farther from such systems, often present materials through seminars. Some programs do not cover rapid rail travel in their curricula at all.

When they were asked to specify their curriculum materials, many of the respondents said they used *Orientation and Mobility Techniques: A Guide for the Practitioner* (Hill & Ponder, 1976) or *Orientation and Mobility: Behavioral Objectives for Teaching Older Adventitiously Blind Individuals* (Allen, Griffith, &

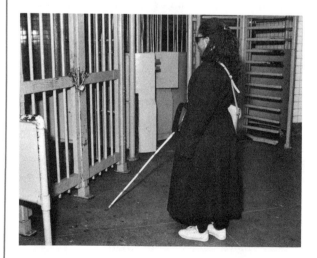

Locating the exit in some stations is difficult, and some exits are open only at certain hours.

Shaw, 1977). Others said they believed that manuals do not cover the topic of rapid rail adequately and that they have relied on presentations made by their own faculty members. When asked about specific techniques and strategies that seemed useful for blind and visually impaired individuals, the respondents described some basic approaches that they use in preparing clients for mass transit travel.

They stress, for instance, how important it is for a blind or visually impaired traveler to become familiar with a station. Self-familiarization using sighted pedestrians is the ultimate goal. An understanding of the concepts of rapid rail travel is a prerequisite and includes knowledge about conveyances, the fare system, lines and routes, platforms, pits (drop-offs from the platform onto the tracks), the third rail, the line of cars, the linking of cars, car interiors, crowds, and door control.

The O&M specialists in the survey believe that much useful information can be obtained by calling the local transit authority prior to taking a trip. Clients are taught how to elicit this information successfully. They are trained to know when it is necessary to solicit aid from the public and how to do it.

The specialists have some set rules for rapid rail travel, which include the following:

1. Use auditory information for orientation. Sounds will indicate the location of the farecard machine and turnstiles; the flow of pedestrian traffic will indicate the path to be traveled.
2. Stay near the wall when walking along a single-track platform and in the middle when walking on a double-track platform and be sure to move with the flow of traffic. As a safety precaution, those using canes should keep their canes in constant contact with the ground and remain in step, thereby enhancing drop-off detection.
3. Once at the boarding location, approach the platform drop-off in a perpendicular fashion, maintaining cane contact with the platform surface. After locating the drop-off, move back and wait for the train, placing the cane in a way that is unobtrusive to other pedestrians.
4. When the train arrives and the doors open, use the cane to locate the opening in the door, reaching in to make certain the floor is present and level with the platform. Draw the cane toward the feet and use it to locate the gap between the platform and the train. The cane should not be extended downward, between the side of the car and the platform, where high-voltage electric collector shoes may be present. Electric collector shoes are devices attached to the train that slide along the electric rail to transmit electricity from the train to the train motors.
5. Once inside the train, locate a pole or a bar for stability while searching for a vacant seat. If possible, try to sit near the doors. When approaching the desired destination, start moving toward the doors before the train comes to a complete stop. Be prepared to localize the sound of the doors opening in order to determine on which side to exit.
6. Locate the appropriate gap between the floor and platform and determine if a step up or down is necessary.
7. Determine the direction to the station exit by listening for the direction taken by other pedestrians.

These routine instructions, as practiced by those responding to the study among O&M university programs, reveal a basic training structure. New methodology needs to be explored further in order to expand the O&M curriculum to include every eventuality that the client might encounter. Relevant material would cover topics such as other methods of station orientation, instructor positioning, more detailed development of O&M techniques, and the choosing of the teaching area and the best teaching times. Emphasis should be placed on how to solicit information, how to utilize different types of sensory data, and how to handle fare systems. Emergency pit and train evacuation procedures should also be part of the training, as should increased information for clients with low vision.

Work has started in many of these areas. From the mobility professional's perspective, it is obvious that much progress has been made in teaching blind and visually impaired persons about mass transit, but much remains to be done.

The Impact of Fear on Blind and Visually Impaired Travelers in Rapid Rail Systems

Samuel S. Hines

Blind and visually impaired travelers have clearly identified fear as one of the major psychological factors affecting their efforts to master mass transit systems. Fear's influence has been confirmed by my personal experiences as an instructor during orientation and mobility (O&M) sessions. Although other psychosocial factors, such as motivation, dependency, self-esteem, and feelings surrounding interaction with the public certainly have an impact on one's reaction to mass transit, fear and anxiety usually head the list.

The influence of nervousness and fear of failure on the individual depends to some extent on his or her psychic structure and personality as well as on environmental and situational factors. Yet there are some standard elements of fear that affect blind and visually impaired persons when they need to travel on subways or rapid rail systems. Whether they have

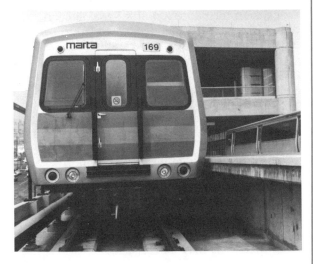

The changeover from an all-bus system to a modern mass transit system has had an enormous impact on blind and visually impaired travelers in Atlanta, Georgia.

a basis in fact or in imagination, these fears must be dealt with by the traveler, the traveler's family or friends, and the O&M specialist.

The Metropolitan Atlanta Rapid Transit System

As an O&M specialist in Atlanta, Georgia, I have witnessed the enormous growth of that city's rapid rail system. The Metropolitan Atlanta Rapid Transit Authority (MARTA) covered a large portion of the metropolitan area with an extensive and well-maintained network of buses by 1975. A few years earlier, a referendum in three counties had authorized the planning of a rapid rail system.

The first portion of that system opened to the public in June 1979, starting with a total of seven stations and a plan for the gradual phasing in of bus service to those stations. The system expanded again and again in the next few years, allowing passengers to go from one end of the city to the other, from east to west and from north to south. Currently, MARTA has 29 rail stations and 32 miles of track and carries 64 million people a year.

During this time, an ever-increasing number of blind and visually impaired persons set about the task of incorporating rail travel into their plans. The changeover from an all-bus system to a modern mass transit system has had an enormous impact on them.

Sources of Fear

The inauguration of rapid rail in Atlanta is relevant to a discussion of how fear affects the ability and willingness of blind and visually impaired persons to engage in mass transit travel. In the case of Atlanta, it was possible to define three different groups affected: those who were used to the buses; those who were familiar with the city's transportation system before they developed vision problems; and those who were familiar with subways or rail systems in other major cities and were then confronted with a totally different system.

In general, anxiety increases when rapid rail is first introduced in a community. The complications of rapid rail add a new dimension of fear to the usual number of frustrations blind and visually impaired travelers encounter with existing systems. Complex station designs are often a cause of fearfulness, particularly since train systems usually have more differences than similarities in their construction and layouts. In any case, many of the sources of fear encountered by blind and visually impaired travelers in rapid rail transportation can be identified.

Time of day can affect a traveler's level of fear. Some stations are busiest and noisiest at peak hours. At other times, they may be so quiet that they limit the ability of the blind or visually impaired traveler to obtain the auditory information he or she needs and expects.

All stations have one area that is—or should be—of great concern to blind and visually impaired rail users: the track area where the train travels. Whether called "the pit" or "the hole," the tracks and the drop-off leading to this area are known and feared. In Atlanta, MARTA designed a 3-foot granite strip to inform blind and visually impaired travelers tactiley when they are approaching this area. This accommodation has caused intense discussion in the blind community. Many feel that the strip is not

Orientation and Mobility (O&M) Specialists

Most rapid transit planners today are fully aware of the need to find physical design solutions that will make rapid rail travel safer and more accessible to blind and visually impaired persons. But public education and training are also necessary.

When a training program for blind and visually impaired users of a transit system is being organized, it is logical to seek the active cooperation of human service providers who are experienced trainers of blind and visually impaired people. Instructors who teach blind and visually impaired people to travel independently in all pedestrian environments, including mass transit, are ideally suited to work with transit authorities.

These instructors, called orientation and mobility (O&M) specialists, are experts at assessing a particular environment and devising techniques that their clients can use successfully to manage that environment. They develop procedures to help clients reach their destinations and, in doing so, to achieve their aspirations. A series of familiarization or field indoctrination sessions is provided that gives blind and visually impaired pedestrians a mental picture of important orientation clues, such as curbs, steps, driveways, sign posts, and fire hydrants. Mental visualization, together with the senses of touch and hearing, is utilized to the fullest extent. The strategies of O&M specialists extend beyond the physical manipulation of the environment for their clients to the vital factors of self-esteem, motivation, and self-confidence.

By virtue of their unique training and experience, O&M specialists develop finely honed skills in dealing with accident prevention and human performance. This makes them effective teachers of independent travel, even in potentially dangerous settings.

O&M specialists, who are certified by the Association for Education and Rehabilitation of the Blind and Visually Impaired (AER), must be trained on the undergraduate or graduate level. They undergo an intensive program of study that includes many hours of learning to travel blindfolded and with special vision-reduction goggles. Although the number of members in the profession is small—there are approximately 1,500 certified instructors—O&M specialists are employed in a variety of settings in every state and in Canada. The *AFB Directory of Services for Blind and Visually Impaired Persons in the United States, 23rd Edition* (American Foundation for the Blind, 1988) lists local, state, regional, and national organizations where O&M specialists may be contacted.

—Mark M. Uslan

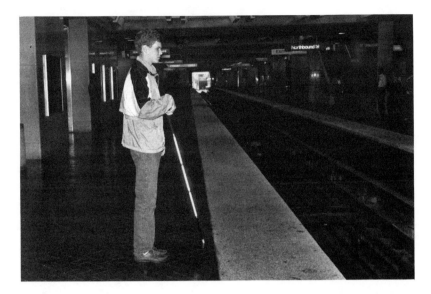

A 3-foot granite strip at the edge of train platforms in Atlanta informs blind and visually impaired travelers when they are approaching the edge.

easily discernible to cane users, although it is helpful to travelers with low vision.

The fast-moving trains are feared by many blind and visually impaired (as well as some sighted) passengers. Some are frightened by the modern technology of rapid rail and by the speeding trains without understanding how they operate. Many who have been riding buses for years are fearful of change and will go out of their way, if at all possible, to avoid riding the trains. Many worry about accidents involving trains and even have claustrophobic fears about being below ground.

Some blind and visually impaired travelers have misconceptions about rapid rail travel and thus are apprehensive about everything in the system. This kind of fear often particularly affects congenitally blind travelers if they have no basic concept of what the system is like. Others especially affected might also include nonindependent travelers who do not go anywhere alone, or those who are resistant, for whatever reasons, to O&M training.

There is a tremendous fear of personal harm or accident, especially in quiet and empty stations in the early morning or late at night. The fear of rape and robbery is also ever present. Crimes occur even in the newer rapid rail stations, where modern security systems have been installed. In relation to such incidents, blind and visually impaired travelers can feel more vulnerable than their sighted peers.

O&M specialists, as well as family members and friends, must accept a blind or visually impaired individual's fear as genuine, empathize with it, and discuss how best to deal with it. The more problems solved with O&M training, the more self-confidence builds, and the greater the chance of overcoming the fear and anxiety that stems from helplessness and an inability to control one's environment.

As they develop concentration, proper cane skills or teamwork with a dog guide, and the ability to interact with others to seek assistance when necessary, blind and visually impaired persons gain the experience and knowledge necessary to overcome fear. Taken together, the proper techniques and skills, enhanced safety, the incorporation of psychological considerations into training, and the sharing of ideas will help a blind or visually impaired traveler make his or her way successfully in rapid rail transit.

References

American Foundation for the Blind (AFB). (1988). *AFB directory of services for blind and visually impaired persons in the United States, 23rd Edition.* New York: Author.

Allen, W., Griffith, A., & Shaw, C. (1977). *Orientation and mobility: Behavioral objectives for teaching older adventitiously blind individuals.* New York: New York Infirmary/Center for Independent Living.

Hill, E., & Ponder, P. (1976). *Orientation and mobility techniques: A guide for the practitioner.* New York: American Foundation for the Blind.

CHAPTER 4
THE TRANSIT PROFESSIONAL'S PERSPECTIVE

Donald J. Dzinski

Without question, there is a growing constituency working in behalf of visually impaired and disabled individuals. It includes those who work with disabled persons, many advocacy groups, and disabled people themselves. And, more and more, it should include members of mass transit systems.

American Public Transit Association

The American Public Transit Association (APTA) represents transit systems all across America. Ninety-five percent of public transportation riders in the United States use the services of APTA members. APTA has over 800 members, about 350 of whom are involved in providing direct services. The others are associate members, planners, consultants, manufacturers, or suppliers to the systems, a broad spectrum of people sharing information and technical expertise. Virtually all the large systems in Canada are members as well; some foreign systems, such as the *Régie autonome des transports parisien* (RATP) in Paris and the Department of Transport in London, are associate members.

For those concerned with the issues of increased and improved services to disabled travelers, we at APTA offer a direct line to transit officials and transit operations, an opportunity for consumers and their friends and advocates to voice what needs to be done for blind and visually impaired and other disabled persons. And, in exchange for information on the needs of the disabled community, transit people need to articulate their needs and their problems.

Although we realize that mass transit authorities need to do more to improve transit systems for disabled persons, we must also recognize some of the issues APTA and its members will continue to face over the next few years, budget cuts being just one of the difficulties in the delivery of service. This does not diminish the fact, however, that the specific, hard problems raised can be tackled and solved. Certainly, APTA, with its unique position in the industry, can move forward to provide help, give guidance, offer coordination, and encourage dialogue among all the people involved.

Our business is moving people and allowing them to get from point A to point B. Doing this successfully means focusing on efficiency, availability, and safety —all at a reasonable cost to the user. It also means attracting a broader market to mass transit.

Sometimes progress seems to take an inordinate amount of time. Although the wheels turn slowly, the transit industry has been following a policy in which local authorities make the decisions concerning any kind of public access or use of transit facilities. Transit authorities are a diverse group, with some systems operating in cities with fewer than 500 people and others in cities such as New York, with 8 million. Our job is to support local efforts with a program that should help transit authorities in local communities make their decisions.

APTA collects data and provides an information-sharing service for transit agencies across the country. It also does research on critical topics, such as demographics, training policies and procedures, marketing, service costs, community involvement, and technological development, and other issues that arise. It continues to pay attention to the provision of transit services for blind and visually impaired, disabled, and elderly persons through ongoing meetings and conferences. In this regard, APTA will want to coordinate its efforts with professional groups and invite them to participate in and sponsor special seminars, workshops, and aggressive outreach programs. It is APTA's intent to solicit the views of representative groups and organizations and to seek the advice and counsel of qualified professionals in the design and content of these programs.

APTA and Local Communities

Under the Federal Urban Mass Transportation Program, the Urban Mass Transportation Administration (UMTA) provides about 80 percent of the cost of capital equipment to systems around the country while local communities provide 20 percent. Given the cost of a new rail system, such as the one recently built in Miami, the 20 percent that comes from local funds is a considerable amount. The size of these costs puts a financial burden on the local community and gives it a significant stake in the con-

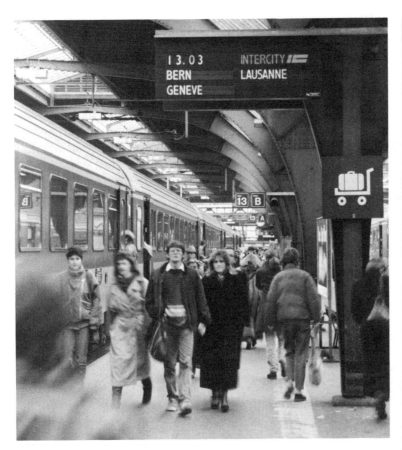

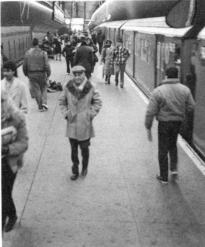

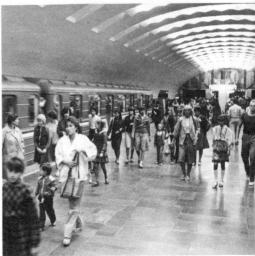

Transit systems throughout the world
serve a large number of commuters.

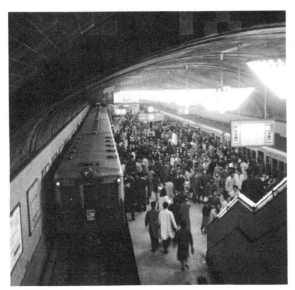

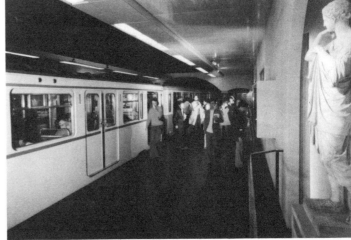

struction and operation of transit systems. Again, APTA's role is to help localities make decisions and choose the systems that will meet their community's needs. Part of this assistance can be in the form of education and training of both operating personnel and the riding public, especially in regard to the disabled community.

The great majority of the general public is untrained in the use of mass transit and unaware of safety measures, so it is important that we reach and educate the public through other means. To do this, APTA can assist local systems in talking to every group representing the public that is expected to use the system, including disabled persons and those who speak for them. It is easier to provide special groups with orientation and training through conferences and workshops than it is to maintain contact with the general riding public through public address announcements or the usual handouts given out at stations.

Safety Issues

Transit officials take a system safety approach to everything. Before a system is installed, a formal and thorough evaluation of any idea or concept delineates both the advantages and the disadvantages. Virtually every safety device that has ever been invented is a double-edged sword. For all the safety elements that each is designed to provide, there is a disadvantage that could cause some significant hazards. For example, the doorbell, which is a safety device that warns riders about approaching when the door is about to close, sometimes works the other way. For some riders, it has become the starting bell! When the bell rings, they run for the doors.

Attention to safety issues is further complicated by the different needs and views of different interest groups. Local transit officials often must deal with varying demands from consumers. They generally recognize, through hard experience, that the disabled community, like the general public, is itself composed of a mixture of groups. Often, what is good for one group may not be good for another. Even within a single group, including those repre-

senting blind and visually impaired riders, mass transit authorities have had to deal with conflicts.

One transit authority's experience illustrates this point. When new cars were designed for its system, two groups representing the blind and visually impaired community were involved. One group wanted a set of beepers over the middle set of doors on each car to steer blind and visually impaired riders toward the door and away from the area between cars where they could fall into the trackway. In theory, it was a good idea. When the safety engineers tried to implement it, however, they found that it posed serious problems, especially because of acoustical complications. If there were two six-car trains in the station at the same time, each car with one activated beeper, 12 beepers would be on at one time! Although the problem was not necessarily insolvable, the second group representing the blind community was opposed to the whole concept. They feel that this system would "make it look like we're so vastly different from the rest of the community that you're drawing attention to us." In many cases, however, we may find that the advantages involved in an idea outweigh other considerations and make it worthwhile.

Training for Access

Access problems should be viewed from the broadest possible perspective. If one looks at the needs of blind and visually impaired people today, for example, one must at the same time study the demographics of this country projected over the next 20 years. There will be a significant shift in the age of our population, and many additional people will face some visual impairment. Mass transit systems must prepare for an increased ridership of blind and visually impaired, disabled, and elderly persons dependent on public transportation.

Specific Needs of the Blind
and Visually Impaired Community

It is imperative to remember that training can help deal with the specific needs of both the general public and the blind and visually impaired community. From a practical standpoint, training may be the only viable solution for making certain that persons using canes or dog guides can determine that an area to be stepped into is actually the door of the train and not the dangerous void between cars, or the empty space in front of or behind the train.

User training is vital to making the system work efficiently and safely for those using it. People must be trained to be aware that certain booby traps do exist and that there are problems that have not yet been overcome. This applies to the general public—those who run to the door when they hear the bell instead of taking the bell as a warning signal—and disabled travelers as well. How many people, for instance, know that the unofficial rule in the Washington, DC, system is to stand still on the right and walk up on the left side of an escalator? Teaching blind and visually impaired people to make the fullest possible use of existing transit systems

will require full cooperation among O&M specialists, their associations, and local transit authorities.

Sensitivity Programs for Transit Personnel
In 1983, the Bi-State Development Agency Training Division in St. Louis embarked on a program to make the agency's bus and telephone operators aware of the special needs of blind and visually impaired and other disabled passengers. Redefining stereotyped ideas about disabilities and embracing this kind of sensitivity program help the industry to identify and accept problems so solutions can be found.

Alternative Public Transportation Services
Training and assistance to increase the utilization of other services by blind and visually impaired people should be considered, too. One should look, for

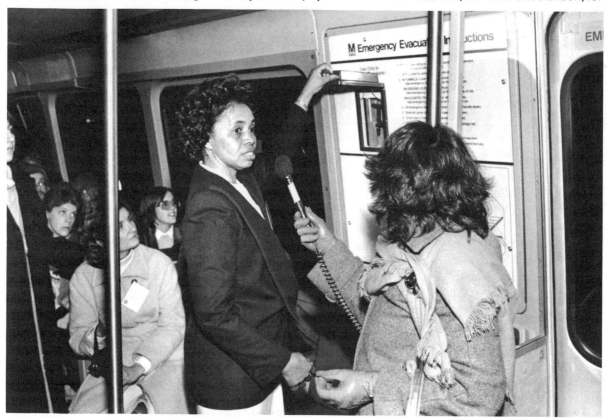

Transit personnel share their expertise with members of the community and professionals in the blindness field through seminars and conferences organized for exchanging information and improving the accessibility of transit systems.

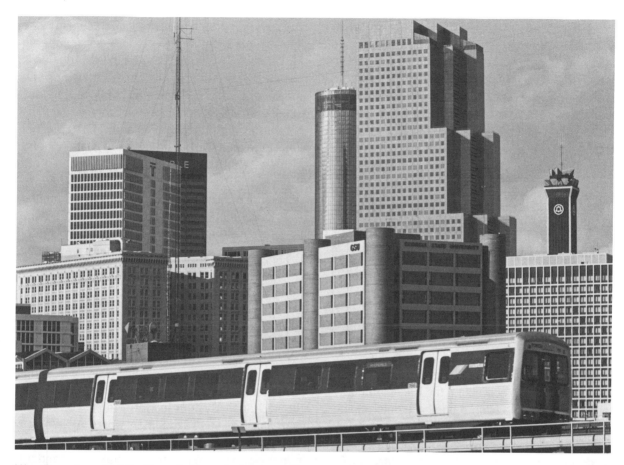

The American Public Transit Association coordinates efforts with local transit systems, such as the Metropolitan Atlanta Rapid Transit Authority, in planning and improving local systems.

instance, at alternative services in public transportation, such as vans and taxis, that are already in place in various locations. There is not enough information on what these kinds of para-transit groups can do. What problems do they pose? What kind of physical, procedural, or training improvements can they offer? In the future, this alternative might gain an ever-increasing market share of the public transit ridership.

Training issues need to be dealt with in as many communities as possible. It is vital to coordinate efforts that will launch operator training and sensitivity programs. Working through APTA's formal safety structures and its bus and rail safety committees, which cover only 30 rail systems but a much larger group of bus systems, APTA and the American Foun-

dation for the Blind, for instance, could coordinate many activities.

Training can bear fruit in many ways. It is a marketing tool, it has a public service function, and it can add to the country's productivity by improving transportation for blind and visually impaired persons who are employed. If these persons have access to public transportation systems—bus or rail—they will get to and from work a lot easier. The result is increased productivity for the whole community.

The Transit Authority and the Community

Making all the physical and programmatic plans for all the riders in all the transit systems in an area involves a great deal of decision making at every level. The question most often asked is, Is the transit authority going to be the one agency with the major responsibility in the decision-making process, in financing, and in implementation? The question seems to imply that complex issues require both an arbiter and an authority—and that would be the transit authority. However, there is a need, as mentioned, for us to reach out more to involved and interested communities and to be sensitive to both their needs and their responses. Every transit authority usually has an advisory board to deal with issues other than general policies. It is difficult for transit authorities to find out who the most appropriate members of those advisory boards should be. This is where the professionals can help. They can tell transit officials whom to talk to and who should sit on the advisory boards. A formal process should be set up to make this effective.

Financial Considerations

Setting priorities is something the transit authority itself has to do, and often money is a determining factor. Everyone knows it does not matter if key features get on the drawing board if the money needed to implement changes is not available. Of what use are safety devices in a system that is not operating because it does not have the money? Usually, it is the general manager who has to make financial decisions and set the priorities. Unfortunately, great amounts of money are not being poured into research and development of improved systems and operations. Yet we are aware that a major effort is needed—and will be made—to secure the proper financial resources, especially from the federal government. This is an important part of APTA's activities, and APTA's success in this area will show its support of professional efforts on behalf of blind and visually impaired riders and other disabled groups for training, programs, and improvements.

In addition to paying attention to financial considerations in the planning of systems, it is necessary to understand the complex aspects of designing and constructing rail and bus systems and, most important, passengers' relationship with the systems. Today, there is a declining number of big, heavy rail systems being built. Los Angeles is the only city currently planning such a system. There are several less complicated, less technically sophisticated light rail systems under way, such as those in Portland and San Diego. These are not quite as expensive as heavier rail systems, and perhaps because of this, the public has had more of a chance to participate in design decisions. Again, getting the right mix of advisers from the community can help ensure that the transit authority's decisions reflect passengers' needs. The plan must also, of course, be operable and financially feasible.

Information Sharing

Some new ideas and improvements are being introduced into existing systems. Some transit systems that were originally built without much consideration for special populations are now being retrofitted. Platform-edge detection systems, especially the test program operating in the Bay Area Rapid Transit System in San Francisco, are an example. When one experiment works, APTA's own safety committee shares that information with the industry as a whole and tries to make it a standard application.

However, we must be cautious about using the word "standard." Coming as they do from different communities, with different opinions, governmental and funding sources, and ways of doing things, transit officials feel that what can be done in one city cannot necessarily be done in another. Innovations and changes are accepted as possibilities or guidelines, but never as "standards."

Without doubt, if 10 safety experts are put in a room and given one problem to work on, they will come up with about 25 solutions. This would produce a broad range of answers that might partially or totally work, and that is what many transit people are trying to do. In addition, a great deal has been accomplished in both operator- and user-training programs to benefit elderly and disabled persons.

Another area in which closer cooperation between transit authorities and the public is needed is in analyzing hazards. It is critical to evaluate the hazards and the problems that could occur if nothing is done about them. We have to look into how often a hazard might arise, because even a minor hazard, presenting itself two or three times a day, becomes a major problem. We need to look for possible solutions. Obviously, the best solution is to eliminate the hazard. If that is impossible, we should look for alternatives, such as changing procedures or installing warning signals. Input from the blind and visually impaired and disabled communities and those representing them would greatly enhance the decision-making process in such cases.

Problems cannot be solved overnight, but the dialogue must continue. National and local agencies working with and for blind and visually impaired travelers must show mass transit officials what the issues are and how we can assign them some kind of priority ratings. APTA welcomes the opportunity to join with these groups in sharing information and evaluating ideas. In addition, APTA can help disseminate information by providing publishing services for the production of materials for groups that want to reach others throughout the mass transit industry. Together, through learning and teaching, we should be able to remove roadblocks that stand in the way of improved transit systems for blind and visually impaired and other disabled riders.

PART II
ISSUES IN RAPID RAIL AND BUS TRAVEL

AS THE BLIND and visually impaired community, transit personnel, and O&M specialists join together to make mass transit more accessible, their focus is on rapid rail and bus travel, the forms of transportation most commonly and widely used by blind and visually impaired travelers. Awareness of the needs of blind and visually impaired and other travelers with disabilities and implementation of new systems that make travel safer and easier for this special population are slowly increasing everywhere. New technical material is being developed and installed. From California, where a new subway platform-edge detection system has attracted attention, to Japan, where tactile systems have been installed in both subways and buses, issues relating to both needs and improvements are being addressed by transit authorities.

Transit authorities are responding not only to new products available, but to advocacy efforts on the part of all those involved and interested in bringing better transportation facilities to the blind and visually impaired community. Communication lines are opening, information is being exchanged, and training and education are producing results.

This section reflects a changing and dynamic mass transit environment. Various issues in rapid rail and bus travel are described, including a rapid rail training seminar held at an international conference on mass transit and visually impaired travelers and innovative equipment being used in various transit systems.

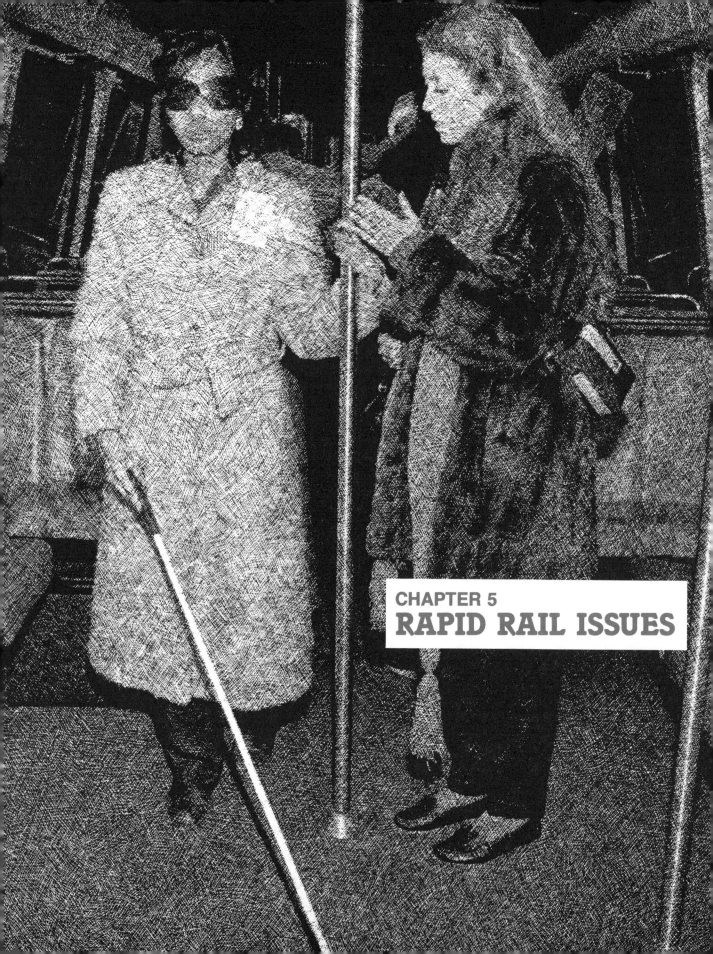

CHAPTER 5
RAPID RAIL ISSUES

The Rapid Rail Training Seminar

Mark M. Uslan
William R. Wiener
James Newcomer

Orientation and mobility (O&M) specialists are the experts who train blind and visually impaired people to negotiate many difficult and different environments as safely as possible in their quest for independent travel. As part of their job, wherever and whenever possible, they provide their students with on-site instruction and practice in traveling in rapid rail systems. The experience of the Metropolitan Washington Orientation and Mobility Association (WOMA) in Washington, DC, and the Washington Metropolitan Area Transit Authority (WMATA) in conducting simulation exercises is an example of what cooperation involving O&M specialists can do to help blind and visually impaired riders. (See "Announcement for an On-site Training Session.")

On-Site Student Training

WOMA and WMATA organized a training session to allow O&M instructors to bring their students to a rapid rail training site—a station that was under construction—where WMATA actually placed a 6-foot track section for demonstration purposes. Each participant went down into the trackbed and familiarized himself or herself with the layout of the rails, the crawl space, and the depth of the trackbed.

The group then moved to a functioning station, and although the students were not able to get down to the tracks, in every other respect, the meeting was a comprehensive training session. Instructors waited in each of five places in the station to give instructions on finding and using farecard machines, turnstiles, and escalators; getting to the correct platform; orienting oneself on the platform and boarding a car safely; and familiarizing oneself with the features of the car. In actuality, this was not an attempt to provide O&M training as much as it was to show competent travelers some of the details and peculiarities of a particular system so that they could travel safely on it.

The real value of such training was demonstrated later when a blind woman who had participated in the program fell off a platform some time after the training took place and extricated herself safely from

---

Announcement for an On-site Training Session

Announcement from the DC-Maryland Chapter Newsletter of the Association for Education and Rehabilitation of the Blind and Visually Impaired (AERBVI)

METRO ORIENTATION

From 6:30-8:30 Sunday evening, June 1, visually handicapped people are invited to a free hands-on orientation to a typical Metro station. Two Metro cars will be on the track in the station, and professional O&M specialists and Metro officials will be present to show:
- How to orient yourself in a station;
- How to use the farecard machines and find the turnstiles;
- How to locate the escalator and platform;
- How to safely enter the Metro car and orient yourself inside;
- How to orient yourself after exiting the car.

Important: This orientation is not an O&M training session and is designed for the independent visually handicapped traveler who would like to become more familiar with the DC Metro system. It is sponsored by the Washington Metropolitan Area Transit Authority (WMATA) and the Metropolitan Washington Orientation and Mobility Association (WOMA).

The orientation is free, but you must call to register first. Also, as the Metro system will be shut down after 6:00, other transportation must be arranged. If this will be difficult, call the numbers below to see if carpooling is possible.

For more information, call Karen Pannell at Metro (962-1481; TDD 638-3780) or WOMA's Dona Sauerburger (858-0138: Voice and TDD).

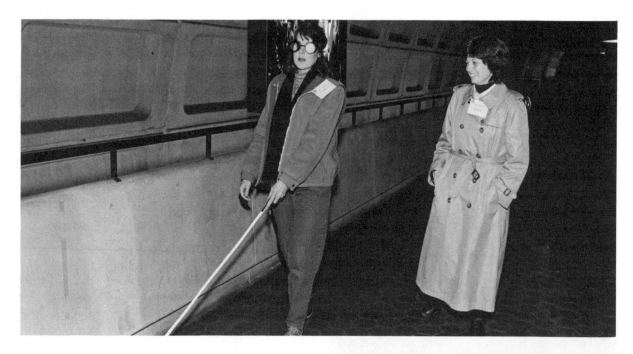

the situation. She was uninjured because she stayed calm and did not panic. She knew what to expect and what to do.

Instructors met both before and after the orientation sessions to share their experiences and evaluate the session. As a result, a comprehensive list of observations and suggestions for using the system was drawn up by WOMA, incorporating ideas from Metropolitan Transit Authority officials, blind and visually impaired participants, and O&M specialists. Copies were made available in print and on tape to serve as a guide and model of the type of material that should be available for all rapid rail systems. (See Appendix 1.)

Training the Trainers

The success of this on-site training program for blind and visually impaired travelers gave the American Foundation for the Blind (AFB) the impetus to take the experience one step further and give O&M specialists themselves actual trackbed and system orientation. Obviously, O&M specialists who participate in such on-site simulation training can be more effective in training blind and visually impaired people in mass transit travel.

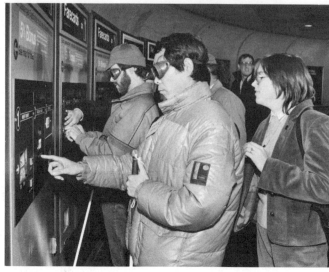

Since normal training for O&M specialists includes blindness simulation exercises, the on-site simulation approach to rapid rail travel is natural for them. Blindness simulation exercises are organized by pairing up instructors. While one instructor simulates visual impairment by using a blindfold, or specially designed vision-reduction goggles to create a visual field restriction of 3 degrees and a visual acuity of 5/200 (20/800), the other instructor takes

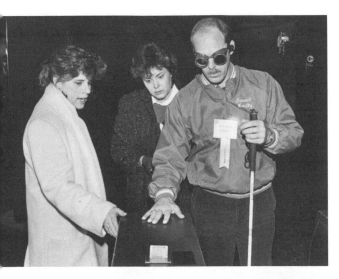

Participants in an on-site training session held in the Washington, DC, Metro system go through the session in pairs, with everyone taking a turn at wearing vision-reduction goggles or blindfolds.

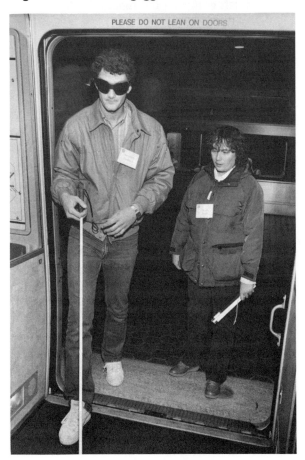

the responsibility of teaching and monitoring safety. At some point during the exercise, the roles are reversed.

In the discussion that follows, a prototypical training event is described. It is based on an on-site simulation program for 25 pairs of instructors planned by AFB in conjunction with WMATA and WOMA. Because the physical layouts of transit

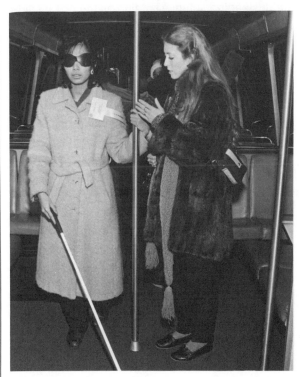

systems in the United States are not standardized, local groups must make their own adaptations. It is important for all those involved in planning on-site simulation exercises to be familiar with the particulars of their own systems.

To begin, participants may be required to present signed liability waivers. They are told in advance to bring canes and blindfolds with them, as well as telescopic devices, if possible. The organizing group supplies vision-reduction goggles and optical aids.

To make the exercise more challenging, a station with a complex floor plan should be chosen. A transfer station with more than one train line and more than one entrance is an excellent choice. Once at the station, the first group of participants is dropped off at one entrance while the remaining pairs start at another street entrance. One instructor from each pair puts on either vision-reduction goggles or a blindfold. Caution must be exercised when using these simulators. When using the vision-reduction goggles, it may at first seem that the amount of vision available is sufficient for travel without a cane, but the environment is unfamiliar and aspects of it are misleading. Intense lighting on the distant side of the tracks may lead one to believe that the edge of the platform is farther away than it really is. Therefore, in the simulation exercise, participants must use canes at all times.

Participants enter the station and the platforms using either escalators or staircases, each group, if possible, utilizing a different type of access. Everyone travels simultaneously to transit cars. Along the route, O&M specialists are stationed at the following locations: the farecard machines, the faregates, the system maps, the escalators, the platforms, and in the trains. At the maps, participants learn how to identify and count the number of stations to their destinations. Instructors are available to provide information and facilitate travel for those simulating visual impairment, directing the participants, when necessary, in the use of the vision-reduction goggles and blindfolds. At the same time, they function as backup safety monitors.

Instructions for the Simulation Exercise Held in Washington, DC

1. Thirteen pairs of students will be dropped off at the corner of 7th and H streets. Before exiting the bus, one member of each pair will put on goggles with a 3-degree visual field. The other will take the role of the instructor and sighted guide.
2. The traveler will locate the entrance to the Gallery Place Station, board the escalator, and descend one level. He or she will follow a walkway to the left and descend to a lower level using a second escalator.
3. The traveler will locate the farecard machines against the wall on the right. Two facilitators will be available to provide basic information. The facilitators will tell the travelers to switch to an acuity lens (20/800) and continue to the faregate. They will also regulate the flow of the participants so that there is enough distance between travelers.
4. The traveler will locate the faregate, where a facilitator will be available to describe the gate. After assisting the traveler, the facilitator will direct the traveler to go to the left and locate the system map.
5. Once the traveler has located the system map, the facilitator will ask the individual to use a monocular to locate the red line at the top left corner of the map, follow the red line to its intersection with the orange line, and count the number of stops necessary to go west to the Foggy Bottom station. The facilitator will ask the traveler to switch to a blindfold and will send him or her to the escalator to the yellow line platform. The next traveler will be directed to use the stairs to locate the yellow line platform. Alternating between escalator and stairs will help reduce any congestion.
6. The traveler will descend one level and will find a facilitator at the bottom. The facilitator will direct the traveler to explore the width of the platform and determine the location of the train.
7. The traveler will locate the train. Next, he or she will trail along the side and locate an open door. After locating the floor of the car and the space between the platform and floor, the traveler will enter the train. The facilitator aboard the train will be available to provide assistance as the traveler explores and takes a seat.
8. At this point the traveler and the instructor will switch roles. The instructor will put on a blindfold and prepare to leave the train.

—*William R. Wiener & James Newcomer*

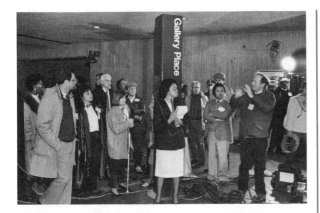

A debriefing session is necessary after a simulation exercise so that participants can share experiences and reactions.

Along the route, the travelers are encouraged to use telescopic devices to enhance their orientation and evaluate the signage. Once the travelers reach their destination and enter the trains, they reverse roles with their partners. The pairs retrace their steps back to the starting point. Approximately one hour is allowed for both partners to participate in the exercise. (See "Instructions for the Simulation Exercise Held in Washington, DC.")

After an hour, everyone reassembles on the platform for demonstrations of evacuation procedures from the train and from the trackbed. (See "Train Evacuation Procedures for Blind and Visually Impaired Mass Transit Travelers.") If the electricity to the third rail can be turned off, a transit official demonstrates trackbed evacuation procedures that could be used in the event that someone fell off the platform. If the instructors are not allowed to go into the trackbed, video monitors on the platform can project what is happening below in the trackbed during the demonstration. Videotaping the entire on-site simulation session is helpful for future analysis and, is important for training those individuals who did not participate. Videotapes play a supportive role in training O&M specialists as well as transit personnel.

The Debriefing Session

A debriefing session for the participants is an integral part of an on-site simulation exercise for O&M

Train Evacuation Procedures for Blind and Visually Impaired Mass Transit Travelers

The safety evacuation procedures for blind and visually impaired or physically disabled patrons are nearly the same as for those who are sighted. The difference is that visually impaired or physically disabled persons would need help or guidance, depending on the severity of the disability.

The following procedures must be followed for blind and visually or physically disabled mass transit passengers in the event an evacuation from the train is necessary:

- A physically disabled person would have to be taken bodily from the train if he or she is in a wheelchair. The chair must be left behind.
- A visually impaired or totally blind person should follow a "lead" person by holding onto a guide's arm, which is held directly behind the guide's back.
- All evacuees should walk along the trackbed to the nearest rail station. The trackbed provides a safer walking area.
- Close attention should be paid to hazards on the trackbed, such as the 750-volt third rail, wet and slippery portions of the trackbed, and any switching devices or other obstacles located along the trackbed.

It is important to remember that in nearly all situations it is safer to remain inside the train and wait for rescue personnel. No attempt should be made to leave a stalled train unless it is truly a life and death situation.

SOURCE: Clementine Newkirk, Safety Training Specialist, Office of Safety and Fire Protection, Washington Metropolitan Area Transit Authority

specialists. The debriefing session is regarded by professionals as a necessary conclusion to a simulation exercise, allowing people to air their reactions immediately, as well as giving them an opportunity to share experiences. A question-and-answer session right on the platform can follow. In addition, time

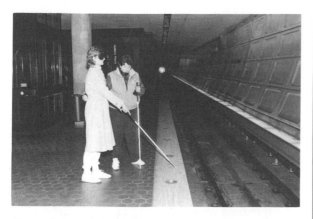

Detecting train-platform edges with a cane is a necessary skill for blind and visually impaired travelers.

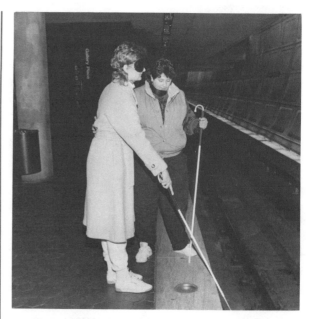

should be allotted to regroup in another place afterward to discuss and evaluate the experience along with the procedures used and to suggest additional approaches. Discussion should include an in-depth analysis of the trackbed evacuation procedures to make certain they accommodate blind and visually impaired travelers in the best way possible. The debriefing session can focus on the following questions:

1. How many have traveled on the platform before?
2. How many have previously experienced low vision simulation?
3. Which part of the simulation experience was most useful?
4. Which techniques were most promising? What works best in what situation?
5. What cane and safety techniques work best on the platform?
6. What kinds of special problems did participants observe in the system?
7. What modifications would participants suggest in trackbed and train evacuation procedures?

For participants, the simulation experience can reveal a host of variables in the environment. It can also point out variables to be considered also in teaching the management of that environment. The experience can trigger an examination of other issues as well, such as, What is the best way to locate a door? Which cane technique should be used under what circumstances? How should the train be approached? How should blind and visually impaired travelers walk along the platform?

O&M specialists using vision-reduction goggles for the first time learn quickly that they must pay attention to lighting when working with their students. They discover firsthand that proper lighting at key points, such as at escalators and farecard machines, is crucial. It becomes obvious to them that certain lights work better than others for visually impaired persons, for example, that translucent signs, illuminated from within, are helpful. The need for increased auditory information is also quickly recognized.

Issues Raised in Debriefing

In the Washington, DC, event, the postsimulation discussion revealed a number of different techniques and points of view. O&M specialists drew on their own mass transit training experiences to delineate the principles that they considered most important. These centered on three dangerous areas: the platform edge, the trackbed, and the space between subway cars.

Shorelining and the Platform Edge

Some O&M specialists teach their students to trail the inner side of a platform's tactile warning strip, away from the platform edge. They feel that following surface textural differences with a cane, or shorelining [detecting the border or edge of a walkway with a cane] lets the student know where he or she is in relation to the edge. Other O&M specialists object to this because of the danger of repeated encounters and possible collisions with pedestrians especially in crowded platforms.

One participant in the simulation exercise pointed out a common problem: "Public interference creates difficulties. You find that people try to grab blind travelers to pull them away from the edge. They think a blind person is in danger, that he's too close to the edge and will fall. The instructor has to be firm about this and make a person trust his or her own skills. Someone who's blind must realize that he or she is in control, particularly if he or she can feel the texture change at the edge of the warning strip and can resist overreacting to warnings from sighted people."

Another danger that concerns O&M specialists involves people who are right on the edge of the platform while waiting for a train to arrive. A blind person walking to the edge could possibly knock a sighted person off the platform. "Falls," said one instructor, "occur because people go toward the platform edge at an angle not perpendicular to the platform." This problem was referred to by still another participant: "When approaching the edge from the center of the platform, there should be something like a wall to square off from, which would allow a blind or visually impaired person to align himself perpendicular to the edge."

Platform-edge dangers and difficulties remain a constant. One remedy would be welcomed by all: If trains would stop at the same place in a station each time, instructors could help their students establish landmarks to board safely.

Trackbed Evacuation Procedures

A demonstration in the trackbed can elicit varying reactions. Some O&M instructors believe that people who fall into the trackbed and position themselves in the crawl space when a train is approaching can get better balance if their backs are on the ground rather than against the wall, as sug-

gested by rail personnel in the demonstration of evacuation procedures that was part of the simulation exercise. However, an opposing view was stated by one participant: "I'd prefer to teach my students to lie on their side, with head, back, and ankles against the wall, lying as flat as possible. That puts more distance between the person and the train."

Everyone agreed that in this situation the person should remain calm and move toward the sound of people who are offering assistance. They also thought that someone who fell on the tracks should not cross more than one rail because doing so could result in contact with the high-voltage third rail.

It is clear that one of the values of postsimulation discussion is to allow divergent dialogue. Dialogue also stimulates constructive ideas, such as one requesting the use of a 12-foot-long model during training sessions to show blind and visually impaired riders exactly how big the space in the trackbed is and where the rails are.

Danger Between Cars

One example cited by a participant summed up a major concern of O&M specialists succinctly and vividly: "In Atlanta, a totally blind woman fell between the cars. She never checked for a floor. She just found an opening." An illustration like this can

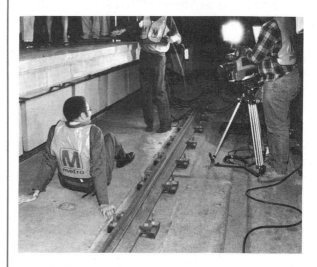

In some simulation exercises, video monitors on the platform project what is happening in the trackbed during trackbed evacuation demonstrations.

produce a number of suggestions. In this particular postsimulation discussion, instructors focused on the need for intercar safety barriers and expanding protection mechanisms. The simulation experience generated new ideas, an exchange of techniques, and hope that changes in the structure of the transit system would be implemented and relationships with transit authority personnel would improve.

Cane Techniques in Rapid Rail Travel

O&M specialists participating in a simulation exercise often want to test and evaluate teaching strategies to be used by blind and visually impaired travelers in rapid rail systems. After the Washington, DC, simulation discussion focused on the value of using a cane on the platform edge, concern was expressed about the probability of a student's being able to detect the drop-off at the platform, even if he or she had good cane technique. One instructor commented: "With the touch technique [or the constant-contact technique in which the sweeping cane is dragged across the surface without it being lifted off the surface at all], I feel a wider-than-normal arc is appropriate, because the traveler might be approaching the platform at an angle. If the arc isn't wide enough, one could step over the edge too easily."

To others, the real danger occurs when a cane user is "out of step," that is, when the cane and the heel of the foot nearest to it strike the floor at the same time. This position can be dangerous when there is a drop-off at the side, rather than in front of the person. Some specialists recommend a longer cane for rapid rail travel. Others believe that a cane that is too long will make it difficult for a traveler to interpret tactile information because it does not really touch down or slide in front of the step he or she is about to take. Still, another suggestion is that, "when they're searching for the train door, students [should] use the cane to shoreline and use their free hand to trail the car as well. That gives double information."

Advantages of Simulation Exercises

Participants in the Washington, DC exercise gave their simulation event an extremely high rating, agreeing that they had gained new insights and perceptions. The concept has been successfully implemented elsewhere, such as by the Bay Area Rapid Transit (BART) system in conjunction with the California Association of Orientation and Mobility Specialists.

For those who have not had the chance before to travel on the platform, the simulation exercise offers an opportunity to find out what it is like and to recognize that, in spite of identifiable problems, the utilization of good mobility techniques and available information can make travel on rapid rail a safe and even enjoyable experience. For the O&M specialist, it is a way of reaffirming the feasibility of teaching travel in this environment. Through simulation, O&M specialists are stimulated to enhance and expand their body of knowledge as it applies to rapid rail travel. Simulation exercises create an acceptance of the reality of problems and provide a forum for exploring possible solutions.

For transit personnel, the lesson is clear: Training blind and visually impaired persons to travel safely in the rapid rail environment should not be overlooked when planning a systemwide public education program. Training O&M specialists through an on-site simulation program offers an effective starting point. O&M people need a heightened consciousness about working with transit authorities to train people and save lives. It is through local associations of O&M specialists that transit authorities can best reach, train, and help blind and visually impaired persons.

Information is what such programs are all about. When O&M specialists have the opportunity to carry out on-site simulation exercises with the cooperation of transit authorities, they can extend the insights gained to their own clients. Debriefing conferences, generating responses such as those described here, are an integral part of the experience.

Detecting the Platform Edge in Rapid Rail Systems

Ralph S. Weule

The ability of blind and visually impaired persons to travel safely in rapid transit depends, to a large extent, on their ability to detect platform edges. Many orientation and mobility (O&M) specialists and transit authorities have tried to combat the hazards related to transit platforms by providing some kind of warning system that will signal a drop-off. In some transit systems, strips of tactile warning tiles have been installed along platform edges for just this purpose.

California's Bay Area Rapid Transit (BART), its Task Force on Access for Elderly and Handicapped Persons, and area agencies have long been concerned

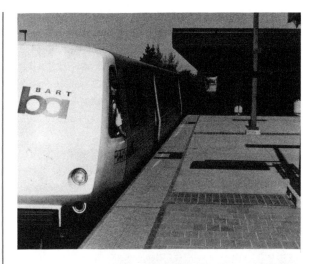

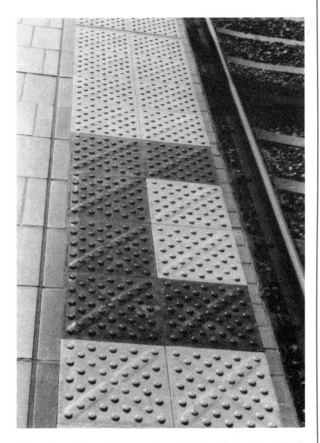

A variety of tactile warning tiles has been installed in many transit systems to help travelers detect platform edges.

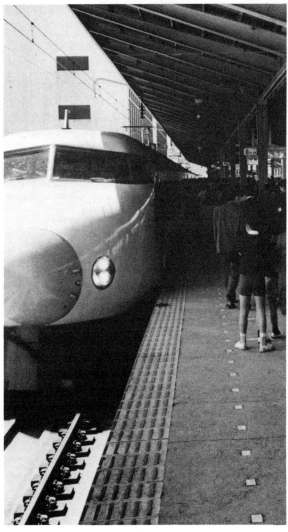

with the 4-foot drop-off from the platform edge to the tracks. BART conducted a study in conjunction with Boston College to assess the effectiveness of a platform-edge detection system and to determine the detectability and durability of several tactile-edge warning systems. (See Appendix 2.) As a result, BART is now embarked on a full-scale application of the findings of the study utilizing tactile warning tiles.

The tiles are made of self-adhering synthetic rubber and have one of two distinct patterns embossed on their surfaces. Detectable under foot, they function as a warning signal of approaching drop-offs and therefore provide clues to direction. They also give off a noticeably different sound from the rest of the platform when struck with a cane, providing audible input for blind and visually impaired travelers. Pathfinder Tiles, the manufacturer of tactile warning tiles used by BART, produces three different types of tiles: the dot or warning tile, the bar or directional tile, and the fan dot warning tile. The specifications for these tiles call for a high degree of resistance to wear, weather, ozone, ultraviolet light, and temperature variations.

Certain problems had to be met head-on as BART proceeded with its research. For instance, installing raised strips or dots on walking surfaces conflicts with basic criteria for walkways and with architectural standards. It could also create a hazard in the form of surfaces on which people tend to trip or fall. But testing and time proved that the concern about the tripping hazard is invalid. BART installed raised materials in four stations, three of which received raised strips based on the Boston College recommendations, and the fourth receiving raised dot tiles. Some of these installations have been in place for over two years and have been crossed more than 50 million times.

After dealing with safety factors, BART had to consider possible maintenance problems. None of the installations showed serious signs of water drainage or slipping problems that could not be solved simply, nor was there evidence of fast deterioration. The synthetic rubber tiles have been installed for over a year in a station that services 12,000 people a day. There has been no evidence of wear. San Francisco is not faced with the problem of snow, and therefore the tiles have not been subjected to salt and sand abrasion. In any case, they are easy to replace.

As in all successful ventures of this kind, the transit authority and the blind and visually impaired community have benefited from mutual cooperation. In California, BART, its Task Force on Access for Elderly and Handicapped Persons, and agencies such as the Living Skills Center for the Visually Handicapped in San Pablo worked together to see improvement over time. The center was able to consult with BART and the Boston College researchers, offer the names of tile manufacturers, and make recommendations regarding colors and patterns. The commitment of everyone involved and interested in better and safer travel for blind and visually impaired persons produced important, practical results.

Some Solutions to Problems Encountered by Blind and Visually Impaired Travelers in Tokyo

Sam C.S. Chen

Some of the concerns about safe subway travel expressed in the United States by orientation and mobility (O&M) specialists have been addressed by rail authorities in Tokyo. With over 11 million residents, Tokyo is one of the most populous cities in the world. Every day millions of people use trains or subways to go to work or school or to go shopping and run errands. The train and subway transportation system in Tokyo has been so well developed that almost everyplace is within walking distance of a station. Trains operate early in the morning and run until late at night, providing convenient transportation for the general public.

Because there are many blind and visually impaired persons in this traveling population, special efforts have been made to enable them to travel safely, easily, and independently. Specific accommodations have been made to facilitate travel and subway use by this group.

Ticket Vending Machines

Tickets for the train and subway system can be obtained from ticket vending machines. The slots for coins, paper money, and credit cards are located at the right top corner of the machines. Four or five rows of round buttons denoting prices can be found in the center of the machines, with labels indicating the fare located immediately above them. Once a button is pressed, the tickets and change are dispensed. At every station, several vending machines have braille labels. Paper money in Japan is also labeled with braille dots and shaped in different sizes for easier identification by blind and visually impaired persons.

Tactile Maps

Tactile maps are installed in some stations, such as Omiya station, which is about 20 miles northeast of Tokyo. On the tactile map, different objects, for example, railroad tracks, entrances and exits, restaurants, and newsstands, are represented by different textures. The description of the texture representa-

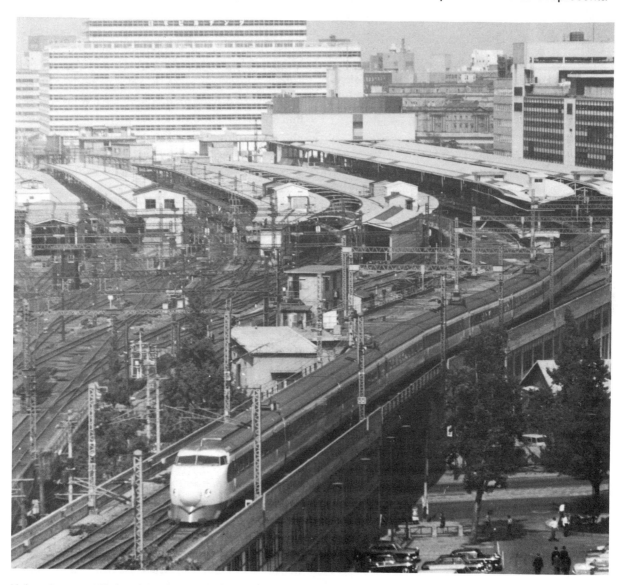

Tokyo has a well-developed rail system that serves over 11 million residents.

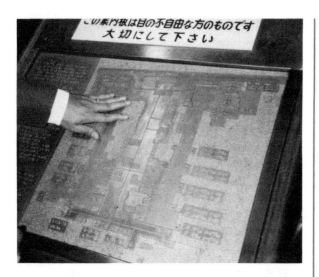

In a tactile map at the Omiya station outside Tokyo, different objects, such as railroad entrances and exits, restaurants, and newsstands, are represented by different textures.

tion is provided on the left side of the map. Blind and visually impaired travelers are provided with instructions on how to identify the representation of the objects, determine their own present locations, and find out where and how to reach their desired destinations. In addition, an audio signal is always in operation to direct blind and visually impaired travelers to the tactile map.

A newer design of the tactile map has recently been installed at Ageo station, which is about 22 miles northeast of Tokyo. The new tactile map contains a three-dimensional model and a series of audiotape messages. Representations of different objects can be found in the middle of the map. For example, a blind or visually impaired traveler can literally feel the model of the stairs that lead to the second floor. There are two rows of switches placed on the right side of the map that provide verbal directions to major public facilities. Each switch is clearly labeled in braille. For instance, a blind or visually impaired person may press a certain switch to obtain the audio directions to go to a recreation center for senior citizens. As in the Omiya station, an audio signal can always be heard to guide blind and visually impaired travelers to the location of the tactile map.

Braille Blocks

Just as they are elsewhere, platforms often are seen as the most dangerous places for blind and visually impaired travelers. In fact, a number of incidents have occurred in which travelers have fallen onto the tracks, causing serious injury or even death. (See "Platform Accidents in Japan," Chapter 8.) In order to prevent accidents, shiny yellow braille blocks, 1 square foot each, with raised dots designed for easy detection by the feet, were installed in stations along a line parallel to the train platforms and about 3 feet from the edge. These can usually be detected by the feet or a cane and can also easily be seen by visually impaired travelers because of their shiny yellow color. Blind and visually impaired travelers are advised to stay behind the braille blocks while waiting for trains. When it was reported that some blind and visually impaired travelers mistook the area between the cars of the train for the entrance to the car door, yellow squares with raised dots were installed on the platform to indicate the exact spot where a traveler may stand in order to

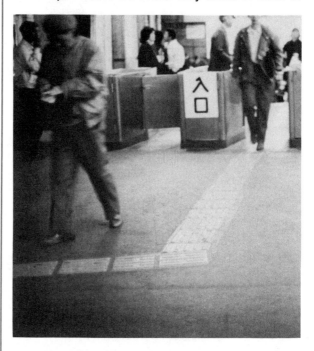

The light-colored path in this picture is the trail of raised blocks that leads travelers from the entrance to the platforms in stations in Tokyo.

be directly in front of the train or subway car door when it opens.

Most people agree that major train and subway stations resemble a maze. For this reason, all stations in Tokyo have braille blocks that lead travelers from the station entrance at the sidewalk to the ticket vending machine area, through the gate, and finally to the platform. Travelers can also trace these braille blocks when leaving the station.

Audio Signals

An electronic audio mobility system that is intended to replace the raised-dot guiding system has recently been developed. The new system utilizes electromagnetic strips and plates that emit an audio signal when touched with a special cane. The system allows a blind or visually impaired traveler to follow the strips to plates that are located at intersections and entrances of buildings, and it can also be used inside to determine directions to individual offices. When activated, the plates provide verbal information regarding exact locations, thus enabling the travelers to reach their destinations.

Inside trains and subways, seats are reserved for physically disabled persons. Like anyone else, blind and visually impaired travelers are often carrying items with them, making it more difficult to hold onto hanging straps for balance. The special reserved seats are thus especially helpful for them too. They may sit there, but are not obligated to do so.

When on a train, blind and visually impaired travelers rely on auditory messages to know where they are. Announcements are made by conductors immediately after departure from a station to inform passengers of the names of upcoming stops. Conductors also announce approaching stops and provide information necessary for transfers.

Taken together, these measures offer important systemwide improvements in the Tokyo rail network. They are designed to increase the safety and freedom of blind and visually impaired passengers, whom they have enabled to purchase tickets, locate gates and boarding platforms, and know exact departure and connection sites. Thanks to improvements such as these, blind and visually impaired

people in Tokyo have been able to become more independent and comfortable travelers.

Light Rapid and Light Rail Systems in Western Canada

Dave Manzer
Kathryn Chew

Our experiences with blind and visually impaired travelers in the transit systems of Western Canada have made us more aware of the need for cooperation among orientation and mobility (O&M) specialists, designers, and transit personnel to make transit systems more accessible to this population. Most of our work has been done in the transit systems of Western Canada, namely, in Edmonton, Calgary, and Vancouver.

These cities use both conventional advanced light rapid transit and light rail transit. Rapid transit refers to an aboveground or underground conveyance that has its own right of way and is used strictly for the rapid movement of passengers. The light rail is a form of transit, generally in cities and metropolitan areas, that uses street trackage and often has its private right of way. The generic term LRT will be used here to refer to both types of systems.

Edmonton's and Calgary's conventional light rail transit systems use lightweight, electrically powered railcars. They run on dedicated railroad tracks and are powered by overhead electrical wires. These two systems run primarily at ground level, although a few sections are underground. The drivers, who manually operate the trains, are also available to provide assistance to passengers as required. Vancouver has North America's first advanced, fully automated, light rapid transit system. The automatic train control center monitors and controls all aspects of the system. The driverless trains run on standard gauge rails along an elevated guideway throughout most of the system. The downtown portion of this system, however, is located underground. Staff may be available to assist passengers.

Edmonton's LRT system was the first to be built. In 1978, a 7.2 kilometer track was opened. Two extensions were completed in 1983. Two more, which are to be completed by 1992, are being planned. The system had a ridership of 680,000 in 1985.

Calgary's LRT, or C-Train, has been in the planning stages since 1966, but construction of the first line did not begin until 1977. It opened in 1981. By December 1987, Calgary had a total of three lines. Three additional lines are planned for the future; however, completion is approximately two or three decades away.

The last three of the systems to be built was the advanced Light Rapid Transit, or Skytrain, in Vancouver. Although Vancouver was the site of North America's first electrified transit system or heavy rail [transit between cities using standard railroad equipment], construction of the Skytrain, which was in the study and planning stages for many years, began in May 1981. The system was inaugurated in December 1985.

Through our experience with these three systems, we have compiled some recommendations and guidelines. They are intended to be useful for designers and transit personnel working to make transit systems more accessible, as well as for O&M specialists preparing training programs for blind and visually impaired travelers in transit systems in Western Canada and elsewhere.

Recommendations for Transit Personnel

- The location and layout of bus stops for transfers between LRT and other forms of transit are important considerations when designing a system. The ideal situation is one in which passengers do not have to cross roads to get to a transfer point.
- Lighting in stations is an important determinant of successful mobility for visually impaired travelers and essential for the safety of all. Especially in underground stations, high contrast colors and nonglare surfaces increase a visually impaired traveler's ability to navigate around obstacles. Indirect daylight is the preferable form of lighting, but where that is not possible, levels of nonglare, artificial lighting must be substantial.

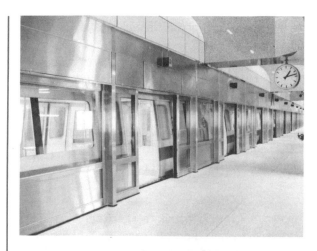

In Singapore, glass partitions that prevent travelers from falling into the trackbed are a unique accommodation for blind and visually impaired travelers. However, the glare from the glass can cause problems for some people with low vision.

- Ticket machines, telephone booths, planters, and benches placed next to walls or railings should demarcate clear, high-volume pathways for pedestrians, cane users, and wheelchair users.
- Signs mounted on walls at eye level are desirable. If signage must be placed in the center of pedestrian walkways, then signs should be detectable by the lower 20 percent of the length of the cane.
- Straight, unobstructed hallways with no blind spots are safe and easy for all LRT users to negotiate, and they are especially safe from crime when coupled with remote video monitoring in all station areas. Elevators that are located away from pedestrian traffic should be monitored to ensure the safety of users.
- All obstacles, such as poles with emergency phones, should be placed where they are easily accessible and out of the way of pedestrian traffic. Benches that are not parallel to the platform edge can cause confusion, and circular benches can be disorienting structures for a blind person. Although oblique stairs are architecturally pleasing, they can be a safety hazard and a source of disorientation.
- Stations with multiple access to the platform level can be particularly confusing to travelers, especially if the platform is of the double-track, center-

loading variety. A single access corridor to the platform level is ideal because it decreases the opportunities for travelers to become disoriented. In the access corridor, stairs and escalators should be side by side. Designing a station in terms of single access is not always possible, however, because of building codes and the large or diverse area that a single station may service.

- All systems provide some signage to indicate the direction of travel of incoming trains, but signs are not as helpful to visually impaired travelers as single-platform access and consistency in the direction and location of trains. Signs indicating the location of elevators represent a similar problem for severely visually impaired and totally blind travelers.

- Elevators should be placed consistently in all the stations within the system. If this is not possible, improved signage should be provided to help guide travelers.

- Tiles aligned in particular ways and slight changes in texture and color have been used to create platform-edge tactile warning strips. These strips must be significantly different in both color and texture from the rest of the platform. They should be wide enough and extend far enough from the platform edge to ensure the safety of blind and visually impaired travelers by giving them enough time and space to detect the edge and move away if they find themselves too close to it. A marked change in texture that may cause pedestrians to trip should be guarded against. Changes in color are useful only when the contrast is visible to visually impaired travelers.

- Clear, unobstructed doorways to trains are preferable to those obstructed by poles or other structures. Many cane travelers have inadequate coverage, that is, they do not swing their canes wide enough to cover their path of travel; therefore, doorways obstructed by poles increase their chances of injury. When poles have been modified for wheelchair accessibility, they virtually guarantee injury for cane travelers, even those with good cane skills, unless protective upper-arm technique is also used.

- Seating provided within cars for people with im-

paired vision or mobility should be near the doors. Wheelchair jump seats ensure greater and more efficient use of space because they are out of the line of traffic and can be used by both wheelchair and dog guide users. Wheelchair tiedowns increase the safety of all passengers should the train make a sudden stop, as long as they are placed clear of pedestrian traffic.

- If intercoms are installed, they should be located so that they are easily accessible to seated travelers.

- Labeling of special seating is helpful. However, labels should be placed at a height that is visible to the traveling public, even when seats that are labeled are occupied.

- Aisles inside the cars should be clear and unobstructed. Handholds should be available at both waist level and above the head as well as adjacent to the doors.

Recommendations for O&M Instructors

- Although it is simpler to train blind and visually impaired travelers to travel in a single-line system, more complex systems can be initially presented in the same manner. For some students, a rote training approach may be useful. Once the student has the necessary skills, confidence, and motivation, the rest of the system can be introduced. Students rapidly generalize their knowledge of a station on which they have been trained to another unfamiliar yet similar station. In those systems in which station design varies, students should be trained at each station.

- When travelers use elevators that are in remote areas and are not monitored by video cameras to ensure passenger safety, it is recommended that they seek either the assistance of transit personnel or some other safer means of changing levels.

- Using the standard touch technique to detect tactile warning strips often does not give cane users sufficient warning of the platform edge. Although the touch-and-slide technique, in which the cane is allowed to slide a few inches along the surface after contact, provides a greater degree of protection than the touch technique, the constant-contact technique, in which the sweeping cane is dragged across the surface without being lifted off the surface at all, is easier for the student to master. It is also more effective as a result of the increased contact with surfaces that it provides, which allows the cane user to detect the platform edge more readily than do the touch or touch-and-slide technique. However, using the constant contact technique can cause the standard half-inch diameter nylon cane tip to get stuck on the rough texture on some platforms. If the sticking of the cane tip is a problem, a marshmallow tip will ensure smoother travel.

- Although clear, unobstructed doorways reduce the number of doorway collisions, they increase the danger of visually impaired passengers' falling into the tracks unless proper cane technique is always used. Some travelers will often check for both doorjambs with the cane but will neglect to check for the car floor. If the space between cars is of a similar width to the unobstructed doorway, the traveler who neglects to check for the floor can fall into the opening between the cars. In Vancouver, a number of accidents have occurred that are directly attributable to such poor cane technique.
- Poles in cars and doorways that have been modified for wheelchair accessibility can be difficult to detect with a cane unless protective upper-arm technique is used in conjunction with the touch technique.
- Often, the public uses the "grab and push" method in assisting blind and visually impaired travelers. The traveler, therefore, needs to be aware of and to practice techniques for informing people about and helping them to use proper sighted guide technique. (For a detailed discussion of these techniques, see Hill & Ponder [1976] pp. 18-19).

Information Sharing

Often, O&M specialists and transit personnel provide different information to travelers. Information sharing among mobility instructors and transit personnel working with the same LRT system will result in the identification of the best safety practices and in consistency of information for students who can apply what they learn to new systems and situations. It will also assist in problem solving and in developing new strategies. In addition, information sharing can lead to the development of materials such as maps and memory aids that are economical to produce and useful on a communitywide basis.

Other areas in which information sharing is vital are planning and construction. Vancouver's accessible LRT is a good example of the effectiveness of preconstruction input from advocacy groups, mobility instructors, and rehabilitation engineers. This can be seen in relation to the issue of elevators and ramps. The debate over the cost of wheelchair accessibility as expensive relative to the small number of wheelchair travelers frequently overlooks the large proportion of the ridership that actually uses elevators and ramps. Elderly travelers, dog guide users, parents of young children, orthopedically impaired persons, and those with balance or stamina problems or whose mobility is temporarily impaired all use elevators. People with orientation problems also use consistent elevator location to assist them in regaining and maintaining their orientation. Obtaining input from representatives of different groups will bring facts such as these forward. Awareness of different people's needs is invaluable for planners and designers who want to create a more accessible system.

Our experience with blind and visually impaired travelers has led to the development of a checklist, the Light Rapid and Light Rail Transit (LRT) Lesson Planning Aid, which is used to individualize an LRT system analysis and lesson design for students. (See Appendix 3.) It allows the O&M instructor to review which skills and techniques should be included when providing instruction for a specific student, whether the student is a rote or conventional traveler.

We hope that the recommendations outlined in this discussion will contribute to a better understanding of the needs of blind and visually impaired travelers. Because it is likely that the needs of blind and visually impaired travelers in Western Canada are similar to those of travelers in other systems, these recommendations are relevant to mass transit systems anywhere.

Adaptations for an Accessible Transit System

Billie Louise Bentzen

From 1980 to the present the U.S. Department of Transportation Urban Mass Transportation Administration has been involved in exploring ways of making transit systems accessible to blind and visually impaired travelers. It has awarded several grants to Boston College to study systematically and propose solutions to problems encountered by blind and visually impaired users of rapid rail transit. A sample of solutions to specific problems are discussed here, namely, telephone information systems, letters and numerals for touch reading, and tactile maps.

Telephone Information Systems

Blind and visually impaired travelers do not have access to as much transit information as their sighted peers, and they are often frustrated by the limited amount of information available to them. Like travelers with unimpaired vision, they are frequently reluctant to solicit information from fellow travelers and prefer to seek out transit employees. However, it is not always easy for them to locate transit personnel. Thus the task of getting information required for planning and traveling unfamiliar routes using public transit is much more difficult for blind and visually impaired than for fully sighted travelers. As a result, confusion, inconvenience, and delay are common experiences for them.

A transit telephone information service is one solution to this problem. In a survey conducted at Boston College (Bentzen, 1989b), 41 visually impaired travelers from Boston, Philadelphia, and Atlanta were asked what types of information they would like to have available via a telephone information service. Table 1 ranks the types of informa-

tion required by travelers in the order of importance assigned to them. The five most desired types of information were name of the exit (stop or station), name of the entrance to the system (stop or station), number of stops to destination (exit), schedule or

Table 1: Transit Route Information Desired by Blind and Visually Impaired Travelers

Item of Information	Number of Subjects Desiring Information	Number of Subjects Considering Information Essential
Name of exit from system	20	20
Name of entrance to system (stop or station)	16	16
Number of stops to exit	13	12
Schedule (or frequency)	13	9
Line designation (name, number, color)	12	7
Description of landmark near exit	11	1
Directions from point of origin (e.g., home) to system entrance and/or from exit to final destination	9	5
Transfer information	6	6
Platform level at entrance and/or exit	6	3
Method for identifying correct vehicle	6	2
Direction on which vehicle will travel	5	5
Direction to turn when exiting vehicle	5	3
Mode (e.g., bus, subway)	5	2
Location of the kiosk	5	1
Distance from exit to final destination	4	3
Intersection and corner on which entrance is located	4	3
Fare	4	1
Alternative routes	4	0
Description of station	3	1
Estimated travel time	3	1
Mode of level change (e.g., stairs, escalator)	3	1
Location of exit from vehicle	2	0
Number of stops to desired exit before/after exit	1	1
Whether exits are announced	1	0
Whether the exit is indoors or outdoors	1	0
Whether there is a center or side platform	1	0
Location of the fare barrier	1	0
All turns (for walking in the station)	1	0

frequency of service, and designation of the line (name, number, or color code). These same five items, in the same order, were considered to encompass the minimum acceptable amount of information needed for traveling in the transit system.

Because of the subjectivity involved in this type of data collection, these results do not conclusively indicate either the full range or the relative desirability of different types of information for the persons interviewed. They are, however, indicative of the cluster of information that blind and visually impaired persons desire to have available via a transit telephone information service, as well as the relative importance of each piece of the information. The responses indicate that the needs of blind and visually impaired persons for information are varied.

An experiment was conducted to determine the type and amount of route-related information that can be remembered for use, as needed, by blind and visually impaired travelers. Thirty-two blind persons listened to route descriptions that included 3, 5, 7, 9, or 11 bits of information that were of the types of information enumerated in Table 1. In 70 percent of all the trials in which they were presented, 8 bits of information were recalled; however, only 72 percent of the subjects could recall all three of a set. Many participants indicated that they prefer to write directions down as someone is giving them. This means that when long instructions are involved, it is important to have a way to control the rate at which directions are given or to have them repeated.

On the basis of the results of the survey, it is recommended that the following information be included for blind and visually impaired persons: the name of the stop or station to get on, the name of the stop or station to get off, and the number of stops between these stops or stations. In addition, the following information may be added to enhance the independence and confidence of blind and visually impaired transit users: the transit line (color code, name, or number), the direction needed to go through the fare barrier (right or left), the direction of travel needed to reach the platform (up or down), the side of the vehicle on which to exit (right or left), and the direction of travel from the train to the exit

(up or down). It is also recommended that the messages in automated systems be repeated so that the directions can be transcribed by passengers for reference during travel.

Letters and Numerals for Touch Reading

Tactile signs have been found to be preferred by blind persons in such locations as elevators, offices, and restrooms in transit systems. The following discussion outlines specifications for letters and numerals recommended for touch reading (Bentzen, 1989d).

Raised characters (capital letters and numbers) meeting specifications of the American National Standards Institute (ANSI) for size (5/8 inches to 2 inches) and height off the base surface (1/32 inches minimum) are recommended for tactile signs on transit properties. Raised characters higher than 2 inches should not be used.

The character width-to-height proportions of the Helvetica type style, which fall under the ANSI standard between 3:5 and 1:1, are legible for touch readers. Exaggerated type styles in width-to-height proportions will definitely be less legible for touch readers. Unfortunately, some raised characters that are exaggerated are in common use. They fit in narrow spaces and may be selected for that reason. Absolute stroke width is a more important determiner of legibility to touch than is stroke width-to-height ratio. For characters 5/8 inch to 1/2 inch, stroke width should be no greater than 1/16 inch. Characters that are 2 inches in height are legible, however, with a stroke width of 1/4 inch. Specifications for stroke width should, therefore, not be stated in terms of stroke width-to-height ratio but in absolute terms.

For raised characters 5/8 inch high that have a stroke width of 1/16 inch measured at the flat surface from which the characters are raised, the shape of the raised profile is a significant determinant of legibility. Strokes that are rounded, trapezoidal, or triangular in raised profile result in characters that are read more quickly and accurately by touch than are strokes that are rectangular. Therefore, the rais-

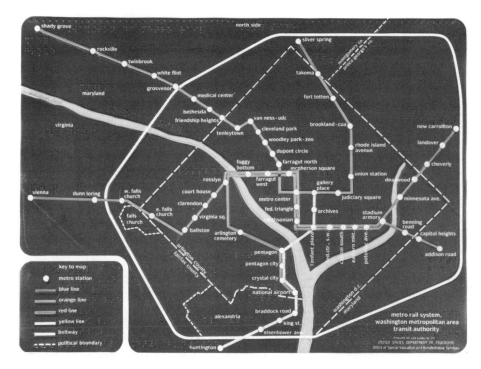

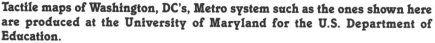

Tactile maps of Washington, DC's, Metro system such as the ones shown here are produced at the University of Maryland for the U.S. Department of Education.

ed profile of a stroke should be rounded, trapezoidal, or triangular, not rectangular. Incised characters meeting ANSI standards (i.e., 2 inches high, 1/4 inch wide, 1/32 inch deep) are difficult to read by touch and therefore should not be used.

Tactile Maps

Research on tactile maps (Bentzen, 1989a) indicates that 77.5 percent of totally blind travelers are interested in using such maps. Transit planners should therefore look for low-cost ways to produce tactile maps for the use of persons who desire route information in this form. Fortunately, it is possible to make transit maps of good tactile quality using "low-tech" and low-cost methods.

Tactile maps can be designed by orientation and mobility (O&M) instructors or by others who have learned the principles of tactile perception and the information needs of blind and visually impaired travelers. Master copies of maps can be produced by the designer or by a skilled craftsperson using a variety of techniques (Bentzen, 1980). Copies of the maps can then be produced by vacuum forming. Many schools or agencies providing services for blind persons have the necessary equipment for this. The maps can include visual graphics and large print as well as tactile information so that they are equally usable by totally blind and visually impaired travelers.

Establishing a cooperative project between the transit authority and a school or agency for blind students can make the cost of designing, producing, and distributing tactile transit maps very low. A side benefit of such a cooperative agreement, possibly contributing more to transit ridership by blind and visually impaired people than the maps themselves, is that the availability of tactile transit maps to teachers of O&M will both aid and motivate these teachers in their instruction of blind and visually impaired persons in the use of public transit.

An alternative to consider is the several facilities specializing in the design and production of tactile maps. Maps produced by these facilities may be much more visually appealing than those produced through cooperative projects and may be equally useful to totally blind and visually impaired travelers, even though they will not necessarily have better tactile qualities. They will also probably be more expensive. Tactile map production facilities are listed in the resource section of this book.

A guiding principle in the design of tactile transit maps should be that using only single, narrow, raised lines to represent the various lines of a system will facilitate rapid reading of the maps, make it possible to contain a maximum of information in a minimum of space, and, probably, result in a spatial configuration that is easier for blind persons to perceive and remember than a configuration displayed in double lines. If single and double lines are to be used on the same map, the double lines should be not more than .12 inch apart; otherwise one side of the double line will frequently be confused with a single line having similar texture.

Tactile transit maps should contain at least the following information: the lines of the system, the location of each station stop in the system, and the name of each station. It is possible to use lines having different textures to represent different lines of a system, in a way analogous to that in which colors are commonly used on print maps of transit systems. Such lines should, however, be carefully selected, and it may be difficult in some production techniques to find more than four line textures that are readily discriminable from each other.

Reports on other solutions and recommendations for a more accessible transit system have been published and are available for use by transit authorities (Bentzen, 1989c; Bentzen, Jackson, & Peck, 1981a; 1981b, 1981c; 1981d; Bentzen & Peck, 1989a; 1989b; Peck & Bentzen, 1987; 1989). The U.S. Department of Transportation does not require transit authorities to implement recommendations presented in these reports. However, the material is available for transit authorities that have the local option to select what is relevant to their specific needs and financial abilities.

Innovations for Improving Systemwide Accessibility

Alec F. Peck

If a whole new transit system were being designed, how would an accessible system be built from the ground up? What innovations might be introduced in order to make the system more accessible for blind and visually impaired travelers?

The answers to questions such as these are in the realm of dreams and visions. When we are unencumbered by real budgets, we are free to envision a public transit system easily accessible to all travelers. New technology offers options that beg to be tinkered with and opportunities that stimulate the imagination.

This discussion will describe two innovations that could be of value to the blind and visually impaired community. Many others have been conceived, but these two were taken beyond conception to the stage of preliminary testing.

Auditory Pathways

One of the major challenges facing travelers in many rapid rail stations is learning or recalling where to go in order to wait for the correct train. When the station or system is new to the traveler, the problem is typically more difficult to solve, requiring the use of maps or signs for most individuals. When the traveler is blind or visually impaired, the problem may be even more difficult to solve, especially if locating the correct platform involves finding a particular area or making a level change, such as going up a stairway or down an escalator. One solution to the problem that is relatively low in cost would be the creation of an auditory pathway.

An auditory pathway consists of a series of electronically programmed loudspeakers located at strategic points in a station. The loudspeakers are activated when a traveler who wishes to use the pathway presses a button at the entrance of the station. Instructions from the loudspeaker lead the traveler to a second location, such as the turnstiles.

The loudspeakers, which are electronically programmed to detect the person's presence, then give the next set of instructions. These instructions in turn direct the person to successive loudspeakers that furnish instructions eventually leading to his or her final destination. The instructions are unique to the station in which they are delivered.

Advantages

Such a pathway has several advantages:

- It can be used by blind and visually impaired travelers to find a destination accurately, even in the absence of other, more familiar cues.
- It can be used to alert blind and visually impaired and other travelers to the existence of obstacles or potential dangers, such as level changes or blind alleys.
- It can be used by individuals who cannot read, such as some mentally retarded or learning disabled travelers, or by children who have not yet adequately mastered the skill of map reading.
- It can be programmed to provide instructions in languages other than English when signaled to do so, enabling non-English speakers to use the system safely and confidently.

The technology needed to implement such a pathway is readily available at a reasonably low cost. Any of several devices can be used, some that require the user to carry a complementary device and others that can be controlled by remote sensors or buttons.

Other Variables

But although the concept of an auditory pathway is intuitively appealing and might at first glance be relatively straightforward, the demands of a noisy, bustling transit environment introduce several confounding variables. In such an environment, how would travelers recognize that a particular message was meant for them? Would travelers benefit from the repetition of a message or from confirmation that the chosen pathway was correct? If a message described a measure distance (e.g., ''The entrance to an escalator is 10 feet ahead''), could most travelers reliably estimate that distance?

Research on these and other aspects of auditory pathways was undertaken at Boston College under a grant from the Urban Mass Transportation Administration (Peck, 1989a). The study was conducted in a laboratory simulation of a real transit environment and revealed several interesting findings. Among them were the following:

- In general, auditory pathways are effective and would probably be used by blind and visually impaired travelers in many stations. Unfamiliar stations and complex stations (whether familiar or not) present special challenges in regard to which an auditory pathway could be of assistance.
- It is not necessary to cue travelers to the auditory messages, even amid noise. Subjects attended to pathway instructions with or without cues.
- Confirmation that one is on the correct path enhances performance considerably.
- Estimating distance (e.g., in response to ''Walk 20 feet straight ahead'') and degrees to turn (e.g., ''Turn right 90 degrees'') was difficult for most subjects, and this type of information is probably not very useful on auditory pathways. Instead, instructions should be given at or near the actual location of a stop, turn, or level change, so that travelers are not burdened with estimating distances in a distracting environment.

Substantial additional research needs to be carried out before auditory pathways can be installed in transit systems. But the fundamental idea is sound, and pathways appear to be a desirable feature of an accessible rapid rail transit environment.

Auditory Beacons

One of the dangers facing blind and visually impaired travelers who use a cane as a travel aid in rapid rail transit is the gap between railcars on a train. Gaps between cars present a serious hazard, especially in crowded, noisy, or confusing stations, when travelers are most likely to rely on information from a cane to determine the location of an open car door.

Travelers who have been taught to use a cane by a qualified orientation and mobility (O&M) instructor in the rapid rail environment should be able to locate an open railcar door reliably. However, when a traveler has not been professionally trained to use a cane in such a situation, or when anxiety, fatigue, or other personal factors lead to an inappropriate use of a cane, the traveler may tap on what he or she believes are the two sides of the doorway opening and proceed to walk ahead into what is believed to be the car but what may in fact be the open gap between cars. Making matters worse, the change in acoustics that is perceived when the gap between cars is encountered may be mistaken for confirmation of the doorway and act as an additional clue that an open doorway has been located.

Several accidents related to this hazard have been reported. The most common defense against this danger is the installation of special gates between railcars that prevent individuals from falling into the gap by effectively removing it. Another solution that is less costly and would aid both blind and visually impaired and normally sighted travelers in determining the presence of a safe doorway would be an auditory beacon. Located immediately above a railcar door, this device would emit an acoustic signal confirming the presence of an open doorway that one can pass through safely.

Like the auditory pathway, the basic idea of a beacon seems relatively straightforward, but it becomes complicated when the noisy and confusing rapid rail environment is considered. How loud would the sound need to be to be heard reliably but not cause unnecessary or irritating noise? What sounds would be perceived as beacons, that is, as guiding devices—rather than as warnings or just noise?

Although many questions such as these need to be answered before standardization of auditory beacons can be accomplished, the basic concept was tested in a laboratory setting that attempted to duplicate the noise and confusion of a rapid rail station (Peck, 1989b). Overall, the experiment indicated that an auditory beacon would be a useful device for blind and visually impaired travelers, that any of several signals could accomplish the desired result without being any louder than the general level of noise in the station, and that the beacon signals tested would be effective at a distance of up to 15 feet, an important feature in the open, sometimes cavernous spaces of a rapid rail environment.

Nevertheless, additional research needs to be carried out, especially on-site research, before final recommendations can be made to transit authorities. But the laboratory results indicate that the idea would probably work and that transit authorities interested in such a system should be encouraged to develop it further.

The auditory pathway and the auditory beacon are two possible systemwide innovations that could make rapid rail transit more accessible. They are also both relatively cheap and use proven technology. If an opportunity to design a new rapid rail environment arises, both these concepts should be seriously considered.

References

Bentzen, B.L. (1980). Orientation aids. In R. Welsh & B. Blasch (Eds.), *Foundations of orientation and mobility.* New York: American Foundation for the Blind.

Bentzen, B.L. (1989a). *Considerations in the design of tactile maps for use by visually impaired travelers on rail rapid transit.* Washington, DC: U.S. Department of Transportation Urban Mass Transportation Administration.

Bentzen, B.L. (1989b). *Enhanced transit telephone information systems to promote accessibility of transit to visually impaired travelers.* Washington, DC: Department of Transportation Urban Mass Transportation Administration.

Bentzen, B.L. (1989c). *Laboratory research concerning tactile warning tiles to promote safety in the vicinity of transit platform edges.* Washington, D.C.: U.S. Department of Transportation Urban Mass Transportation Administration.

Bentzen, B.L. (1989d). *Specification for letters and numerals for touch reading.* Washington, DC: U.S. Department of Transportation Urban Mass Transportation Administration.

Bentzen, B.L., Jackson, R.M., & Peck, A.F. (1981a). *Solutions for problems of visually impaired users of rail transit.* Vol. 1 of *Improving communications with the visually impaired in rail rapid transit systems.* Washington, DC: U.S. Department of Transportation Urban Mass Transportation Administration.

Bentzen, B.L., Jackson, R.M., & Peck, A.F. (1981b). *Information about visual impairment for architects and planners.* Vol. 2 of *Improving communications with the visu-*

ally impaired in rail rapid transit systems. Washington, DC: U.S. Department of Transportation Urban Mass Transportation Administration.

Bentzen, B.L., Jackson, R.M., & Peck, A.F. (1981c). *Techniques for improving communications with the visually impaired users of rail rapid transit systems.* Vol. 3 of *Improving communications with the visually impaired in rail rapid transit systems.* Washington, DC: U.S. Department of Transportation Urban Mass Transportation Administration.

Bentzen, B.L., Jackson, R.M., & Peck, A.F. (1981d). *Selection of tokens and orientation of farecards by visually impaired users of rail rapid transit.* Vol. 4 of *Improving communications with the visually impaired in rail rapid transit systems.* Washington, DC: U.S. Department of Transportation Urban Mass Transportation Administration.

Bentzen, B.L., & Peck, A.F. (1989a). *In-transit research concerning tactile warnings to promote safety in the vicinity of transit platform edges.* Washington, DC: U.S. Department of Transportation Urban Mass Transportation Administration.

Bentzen, B.L., & Peck, A.F. (1989b). *Tactile warnings to promote safety in the vicinity of platform edges: Labora-* *tory testing of pathfinder tiles vs. "corduroy."* Washington, DC: U.S. Department of Transportation Urban Mass Transportation Administration.

Hill, E., & Ponder, P. (1976). *Orientation and mobility techniques: A guide for the practitioner.* New York: American Foundation for the Blind.

Peck, A.F. (1989a). *Considerations in the design of an auditory beacon for use in rail rapid transit.* Washington, DC: U.S. Department of Transportation Urban Mass Transportation Administration.

Peck, A.F. (1989b). *Enhancing access to rail rapid transit via an auditory pathway.* Washington, DC: U.S. Department of Transportation Urban Mass Transportation Administration.

Peck, A.F., & Bentzen, B.L. (1987). *Tactile warnings to promote safety in the vicinity of transit platform edges.* Washington, DC: U.S. Department of Transportation Urban Mass Transportation Administration.

Peck, A.F., & Bentzen, B.L. (1989). *Validation of techniques improving communication with the visually impaired in rail rapid transit.* Washington, DC: U.S. Department of Transportation Urban Mass Transportation Administration.

INFORMATION FOR TEACHING VISUALLY HANDICAPPED TRAVELERS IN METROPOLITAN WASHINGTON, DC'S, RAPID RAIL TRANSIT SYSTEM

APPENDIX 1

Compiled by the Metropolitan Washington Orientation and Mobility Association

(A Division of the DC-Maryland Association for Education and Rehabilitation of the Blind and Visually Impaired)

Mobility Instructors, Metro Representatives, and Riders:

The following information is a composite of notes written by mobility instructors, Metro officials, and blind and visually impaired persons regarding the Metrorail system as it relates to visually handicapped riders. Additions, deletions, suggestions, and corrections are welcome and encouraged. The information is being revised regularly. An audible copy is also available on cassette. Please mail any input, questions, or requests for copies to: Linda Sussman, 3815 Williams Lane, Chevy Chase, MD 20815.

Introduction

This handout is meant for mobility instructors to use when orienting a client to the Metrorail System in Washington, DC, and the metropolitan area. Because each station is different, it does not attempt to describe any details of the Metro system, but does point out characteristics that can be found in many of the stations. It contains teaching suggestions that should be modified as the instructor sees fit.

Metrorail Information

(202) 637-7000 Route information, brochures,
(TDD 638-3780) timetables, locations where reduced farecards can be purchased. 6:00 AM to 11:30 PM, seven days a week.

(202) 962-1245 Handicapped Assistance Office
(TDD 628-8973) (for information on Handicap Identification Cards and locations where reduced farecards can be purchased).
(202) 637-1328 Consumer Assistance Office (representatives handle complaints, commendations, and other more general inquiries. They can also mail brochures and timetables).
(202) 962-1195 Lost and Found.
(202) 962-2121 Metro Transit police (24-hour service).

ID Cards

ID cards must be obtained prior to purchasing handicapped reduced farecards for Metrorail. These may be obtained, free of charge, at the main office of the Washington Metropolitan Area Transit Authority (WMATA). The office is located at 600 Fifth Street, NW, Washington, DC 20001, across from the Judiciary Square Metro station. Nine other sites are available for obtaining ID cards by appointment only. The application for ID cards can be obtained from the Handicapped Assistance Office and must be completed by a doctor in order to verify the visual handicap.

The special senior citizen/handicapped farecards may be purchased with an ID card at all Metro sales outlets, some area banks, and other facilities. To find the closest facility, call the Route Information telephone number or the Consumer Assistance Office for a current list.

Fares vary according to distance traveled. The reduced handicapped fare is set at one-half the rush hour fare at all times, rounded down to the nearest 5 cents, not to exceed 80 cents. Reduced farecards can be purchased in increments of $3 and $8.

Mobility instructors can be classified as an attendant to receive reduced fares when working with a client. To obtain an Attendant Identification Card, a letter must be written on agency stationery and signed by the personnel involved with client travel. The instructor can then obtain the ID card at the main WMATA office or at one of the nine other sites by appointment only. The Attendant ID entitles the instructor to the same fare as the blind rider when they are traveling together on the Metro system.

Attendant status may also be obtained by individuals such as family members and teachers who travel with a blind rider if that person is unable to travel independently. Call the Handicapped Assistance Office for further information.

Low Vision Note: Large, poster size maps of the Metrorail system—the same as those used within the station—are available. These can be purchased in person from the WMATA office for $10, or send a check or money order for $13 to Metro Maps, WMATA, 600 Fifth Street NW, Washington, DC 20001.

Farecard Machine

It is now possible to purchase a handicapped reduced farecard at the farecard machine. Purchasing a farecard at the farecard machine entails three steps, moving from the left side of the machine to the right side. Buttons are raised. The print is incised on the button and can sometimes be discerned. They are not marked in braille.

You can either purchase a new farecard or add money to an old farecard, but you cannot get a refund from an old farecard. If purchasing a new card, begin with the first step below; if upgrading an old farecard, insert it first in the proper slot, then begin with the first step below.

The first step is to insert money. The machine will take $1 and $5 bills. Some of the newer machines will take ten and twenty dollar bills. The rider can determine by touch whether a specific machine will take larger bills or not because the slot in which old

farecards are inserted is shaped differently on the farecard machines that accept ten and twenty dollar bills than on the older farecard machines.

Bills must be inserted with the President's head facing up—the top of the head facing to the right and the lower part of the head facing left. If not facing the designated direction, the bill will be returned. The bill should then be turned in a different direction and reinserted until it is accepted by the machine. Occasionally the machine will return a bill that has been properly inserted, usually because it is wrinkled or torn. Folding a wrinkled bill lengthwise and then unfolding it will sometimes make the bill more acceptable to the machine. Machines are sometimes broken. This would be indicated by red or green lettering lit up above the buttons. The station attendant should be contacted if the machine continues to fail to respond. Coins might be recommended, due to the sensitive nature of the farecard machine with respect to bills. The rider should have all the necessary money prepared before using the farecard machine because the machine will return money deposited if no action occurs after a specific amount of time.

The second step allows the rider to decide the value of the farecard. There are two add/subtract buttons. The left button will add or subtract in increments of $1; the right button will add or subtract in increments of 5 cents. Pressing the top of the button will designate addition; the bottom of the button will designate subtraction. When pushed with a quick, light motion at the bottom or top edge, these buttons make clicking noises that can be counted to determine the digital number being displayed on the machine. If the button is pushed near the center it may not register. If the button is held down too long, it will register repeatedly until it is released.

Low Vision Note: The amount being registered is displayed as red digital numbers above the add/subtract buttons. The value of the old farecard is also displayed here when it is inserted.

The third step entails pushing a square button located toward the right of the machine. The farecard is automatically ejected from a slot to the right of the button. On the newer farecard machines—those that accept $10 and $20 bills—the slot next to the square button is closed off. The farecard is ejected from a slot below the square button on these newer machines. The slot that is located below the square button is also where old farecards can be inserted in order to be upgraded on both the old and newer farecard machines.

From Farecard Machines to Faregates

To determine the location of the faregate from the farecard machine area, the rider can:

1. Listen to people entering the faregate to establish its location.
2. Use any wall as a guideline that will eventually lead (in the form of a wall or a railing) to a faregate.

The tiled floor of the Metrorail stations is extremely slippery when wet. On days when it is wet outside, the tile usually becomes wet, especially close to the entrance of the station. Sometimes there are leaks in the ceiling of the station that also cause the floor to become wet. Yellow plastic signs that say "Caution-Wet Floor" are often placed in the wet areas.

Kiosk

The kiosk is usually located next to or between faregates. An attendant is often inside the kiosk to answer questions and distribute maps and time-tables. On the outside of the kiosk, at about shoulder level, is a speaker for talking directly to the attendant. When the attendant is not there, he or she may be somewhere else in the station or may be out during lunchtime.

Two stations, Gallery Place and McPherson Square, have phones on the outside of the kiosks. This was part of an experimental program where, on weekends, one station attendant is responsible for both mezzanines in each station.

Faregate

Each faregate may sometimes be an entrance or sometimes an exit, depending on the time of day. This can be determined by attempting to insert the farecard. It will be rejected if the rider is entering in the wrong direction. There are usually two lights on the front side of the vertical post of the faregate. The top light is red and indicates "no entrance." The bottom light is green and designates the correct entrance. When there is only one light on the post, it indicates a faregate that cannot be entered because it works only in the direction opposite to the rider's current line of travel. The slight difference in heat may be used by some riders to feel which light is on.

Low Vision Note: Colored lights on the vertical posts of faregates and lights at floor level indicate the location of the faregates.

With the vertical post to the right, the rider inserts the farecard in the slot at the front of the post. The farecard will be returned to the rider. It can be found by sliding the right hand along the top of the faregate, which contains a slot from which the farecard is ejected. The rider should be reminded to check for the returned farecard when passing through a faregate.

The farecard has a small orientation hole that should be in the upper left-hand corner when being inserted into the faregate. This serves to place the card's magnetic strip in the proper position so that it can be read by the faregate.

Gates are programmed to accept a card purchased from the farecard machine only if it has at least the base fare upon entry. Discounted farecards will be accepted regardless of the remaining fare as long as they have at least 5 cents of remaining value.

Farecards will not be accepted or will be returned by the faregate without opening the barrier if (1) the remaining value of the card is not adequate, (2) the machine is not working correctly, (3) the card is inserted incorrectly, or (4) the rider is entering a faregate that is programmed for traffic from the opposite direction. The rider should consult the attendant for advice if there is any question about the use of the faregate.

When there are two sets of gates, each faces a different side of the track, but the rider can get to both sides using either set of gates.

Bus Transfer Machines

Bus transfers must be obtained at the boarding station before getting on the train. They will not be accepted on the bus if obtained after exiting the train. Transfers are valid for two hours from the time of purchase. They will either eliminate or reduce bus fares, depending on the distance traveled.

Bus transfer machines may be found before getting on the escalator that takes the rider to the train platform level. They are sometimes located next to those escalators or the addfare machines. Their location is not consistent.

A button on the front of the bus transfer machine is pushed and the transfer is ejected. A buzzer will sound when the transfer is ejected.

Escalators and Elevators

Standard operating procedures have been established for each station so that the escalators should be operating in the same direction each day. However, when there are mechanical problems, changes in direction or the stopping of escalators is sometimes necessary. Therefore, the rider should always check the moving handrail to verify the direction of the escalator before stepping onto it. Escalator noises sound louder the farther below ground level they are and are therefore sometimes more easily located audibly within an underground station.

Low Vision Note: In most cases there is a light close to the ground, beside the escalator rail. A green light indicates that the escalator is moving in the direction of the line of travel. A red light indicates that it is moving in the opposite direction. Riders should travel single file on the right side of the stair when using the escalator. This is a courtesy, since people frequently pass on the left side.

Most elevators are self-service types, requiring no interaction with the station attendant. The exceptions are those that completely bypass the mezzanine and the fare collection area. In these cases, special fare collection equipment has been installed, which, when working properly, will still allow the rider to use the elevator, in conjunction with a farecard, without any interaction with the station attendant. The location of the elevators is not consistent. Metro's information office can give details regarding the location of the elevator when contacted beforehand. Elevator buttons are labeled in braille. If the

elevator is not on, push the round call button outside of the elevator located to the right of the elevator door. Elevator use can be frustrating because the attendant does not always respond to the call button in order to turn the elevator on. If the attendant does not respond to the call button, push the button labeled in braille and in print "Press to Talk" to reach the attendant. Unless out of order, most elevators remain on throughout the service day.

Platforms

There are two types of platforms: the central or island platform [double-edged platform] and the side platform [single-edged]. Most stations will be either a side platform or a central platform station, but both types of platforms can be found at bilevel transfer stations (where two lines intersect). At these stations, such as Metro Center, Gallery Place, and L'Enfant Plaza, the upper level is a side platform and the lower level is a central platform. There are also split-level stations at merge and bifurcation points such as Rosslyn and Pentagon. The following description of central and side platforms does not apply to split-level stations.

A central platform is located between the two sets of tracks. When one arrives on the platform from the escalator, the tracks on the right will be for the trains running in the same direction that the rider is facing. The tracks on the left will be for the train running in the opposite direction. When the rider faces either track, a train entering the station will be coming from the right when the train is operating correctly. Exiting passengers will leave the train from the doors on their left, assuming that they are facing toward the front of the train. A train entering a station with a central platform at the end of a line, however, may come from the right or the left and arrive at either side of the platform.

A side platform station is one in which both sets of tracks run between the two platforms. When one faces the tracks on a side platform, the train will be coming from the left when the train is operating correctly. Exiting train passengers will leave the train from the doors on their right, assuming that they are facing toward the front of the train. Getting from one side of the platform to the one across the tracks (e.g., to get from the platform for the east-bound train to that for the west-bound train) necessitates going up or down escalators, then crossing over or under the tracks, and finally returning to the original train platform level.

There are two ways to determine if a platform is a side or a central platform: (1) note from which direction the train is moving on the closest track, or (2) walk from one platform edge to either the other platform edge (indicating a central platform) or to the barrier placed about a foot in front of the wall (indicating a side platform). These rules do not apply to split-level stations.

Warning: When trying to determine from which direction a train is coming or when listening for the approach of a train while waiting at a side platform, be sure that the train heard is actually on the closest track. A train that is farther away may be so loud that it is mistakenly thought to be closer than it is.

A rider who is on a train and passes a destination needs to exit the train and get on the train going in the opposite direction to return to the desired stop. It is easier to get off at a central platform, cross the platform, and immediately locate the opposite track than to get off at a side platform, where it is more difficult to get to the opposite track.

Platform Orientation

Having entered the platform from the escalator, the rider is usually facing parallel to the tracks and will probably be approaching the midpoint of the platform. If he or she continues to walk along the platform, the rider will often locate more escalators to enter and exit from the platform. The rider should note his or her location on the platform upon boarding the train because he or she may get off at the destination station at approximately the same place in relation to the midpoint of the platform. This does not necessarily predict the escalator location at the destination station. Escalators on central platforms are not positioned in the same relationship to the platform in all central platform stations. Side platform escalators are positioned differently than central platform escalators.

When trains enter the station, they stop with the train centered at the midpoint of the platform. There are usually six cars to a train, though some stations have trains with four cars during off-peak hours. Eight-car trains are used during extended service periods when there is extremely large Metro usage due to special occasions such as the Fourth of July. In order to board the train, the rider may have to walk toward the midpoint of the station to locate a train car. If a train has arrived while the rider is approaching the waiting area, he or she can judge from its sound how far along the platform will be best to wait for the next train.

After exiting the train, the rider will generally be in about the same relationship to the destination station as the original station. If the middle of the station had been on the right upon entering the train, it will be on the left upon exiting the train. Preplanning to determine from which side of the station to exit in relation to the train direction is encouraged.

Platform Landmarks

Benches, billboards, and trash cans are located parallel to the tracks in the center of a central platform. These landmarks are located along the barrier next to the wall on a side platform. Round cement columns are also sometimes found on the platforms. These are support beams and are not consistently placed.

When approaching the back of the escalator, the rider will contact a railing designed to prevent the rider from colliding with the underside of the escalator. This railing can be followed in the direction of the escalator sound to locate the front of the escalator.

Low Vision Note: Dark metal pillars located next to each track indicate the destination of the train that arrives at the designated track. Sometimes two sides of one pillar are used to indicate the destinations of different tracks, with an arrow pointing in the direction of the designated track. The print on these pillars is at eye level and of contrasting color.

There is a narrow strip of cement with lights imbedded in it at the edge of the platform, which serves as a warning strip. It has a slightly contrasting texture to the tile surface of the platform, but this is difficult to detect using the touch technique with the cane. It is more easily detected by keeping one's feet in contact with the ground and sliding the cane to each side instead of tapping it.

Low Vision Note: The lights imbedded in the cement strip will flash on and off when the train is about to enter the station. These lights are quite dim and should not be mistaken for the brighter lights that are located on the tracks themselves or across the tracks.

Training Suggestion: Walk at a slower pace and keep cane in contact with the floor (sliding) when walking on the platform in order to better detect drop-offs and texture changes.

Tracks

There are three rails parallel to the platform for each train. The third rail, farthest from the platform, is the source of 750 volts of electricity. It is partially covered with an arched-shaped coverboard. The other two rails can also be conducting electricity, depending on how far away the train is from the station. The train will be conducting electricity from the third rail to the other two. The closer the train is, the more electricity will be flowing through the two closer rails.

Warning: When orienting someone to the tracks, do not touch the tracks with a metal cane because it will act as a conductor of the electricity.

The platform overhangs the track area in the stations, creating a crawl space that is large enough for a person to lie in safely next to the wall, away from the tracks. It is about 3-4 feet deep. The platform is about 5 feet above the track area and is therefore too high for many people to climb back onto independently.

The crawl space can be felt from the platform by kneeling at the edge of the platform and reaching underneath it with the cane as an aid in an initial orientation situation. This should be done only under controlled circumstances.

There are train connector paddles on both sides of the cars that always have electricity running through them. Therefore, when orienting someone

to the system, make sure he or she does not use a metal cane to reach down between the side of the car and the platform. Also for this reason it is necessary to emphasize the importance of staying as far away from the car as possible when lying inside the crawl space.

A rider who falls down to the track area should:

1. Listen for the sounds of the people on the platform (remember the relationship of the electrified third rail to the platform).
2. Roll under the platform overhead immediately.
3. Contact the wall of the crawl space.
4. Lie down as close to the wall as possible, making oneself as small as possible against the platform wall of the crawl space.
5. Holler for help.

Entering the Train

To locate the door opening:

1. Listen for the sound of the door operating.
2. Listen to the people exiting and entering.
3. If there are no other clues, walk toward the car, contact it, and turn to trail with the cane along the edge of the car at least 4 inches off the ground (the floor of the car is a little higher than the platform) until an opening is located.

Low Vision Note: Look for the light of the open door that extends lower than the light of the windows.

The train operator is able to see along the side of the train and should be checking along the platform edge. The operator is in control of the bell and doors.

At some stations the track is shared by trains from two different routes (each named with a different color), so the rider needs to identify on which route (i.e., which color line) the train is. On the outside of each train car above the windows, and on the front of the first car, is a sign that identifies the color of the line and the final destination of the train. Some of these signs are coded, and some are digital displays. The coded signs are sometimes not illuminated and are therefore difficult to see. The contrast on the digital signs is very poor, and they are also difficult to see. There is a degree of error in this system in that sometimes the incorrect destination and/or color are displayed. The operator will sometimes be heard to announce the color of the train line and the train's destination. This information is not always audible, and the rider must often rely on sighted assistance to identify which train is currently on the track.

A two-tone chime will ring once immediately before the doors close. Step back when the chime rings and wait for the next train. The trains are designed such that they cannot move unless all doors are closed properly. Hence, if a person is caught in the doors, the doors will have to be recycled and cleared of the obstruction before the train can proceed.

Warning: Before entering the door opening, make sure there is a floor there! If not, the rider may have located the space between the cars and must continue along the train until the doorway is located. If the rider falls between the cars, it is important to get under the platform overhang immediately, especially if the chimes are signaling that the train is about to leave the station. See the section on "Tracks."

While stepping into the car, it is possible to get one's heel stuck in the space between the edge of the platform and the floor of the car. Always step with the foot forward, not sideways, so as not to let the whole foot get stuck in the space. To avoid getting the front wheels caught in the space, clients in wheelchairs or with strollers can enter with the back wheels first or have the front tipped up to lift the front wheels over the space.

Train Cars

There are three doors on either side of the car. Each is across the aisle from another door, with two metal strips on the floor going from the side of each door to the side of the door across the aisle, near the metal strips. There is a pole on each side of the middle door and on one side of the doors near the end. When walking along the aisle to exit, these strips and poles are good landmarks for finding the doors.

Seating for senior citizens and handicapped persons is located immediately to the right or the left of each door and is designated as such by a plaque on the wall above the seats. All seats face toward the front or the rear of the train, except the seats on either side of the doors (including the handicapped seating), which are facing the center aisle. On some train cars there are no seats facing the aisle in order to provide places for wheelchairs and more standing room.

There are doors at either end of the cars to connect the cars. These are to be used by Metro personnel only or in an emergency for evacuating the cars. To the left of the end car doors, at about shoulder level, is usually a protruding emergency call box that has the identification number of the car printed on it. To call the train operator in case of an emergency, press the button and begin to speak immediately. Explain the problem and identify the car number. The operator will not speak until spoken to. Identify the problem so that the operator will know immediately that the call is not a practical joke.

Low Vision Note: A red light goes on where the button is located when the operator is listening. Beneath the window of the doors at the ends of the car is also written the car's identification number in large black letters.

The names of the stations are written in large white letters on black signs that are hung on the walls of the stations. When sitting next to the window on the right side of the train, the rider is closer to the wall at a central platform and closer to the dark pillars with the station name in large white letters at a side platform. It is therefore sometimes easier to spot and discern the station name from this position on the train.

Exiting the Train

The name of the next station is announced soon after the train leaves the preceding station. This allows the rider time to prepare to get off when the car stops. The train operator will announce the station name and on which side the door will open, assuming the rider is facing the same direction the train is moving. These announcements are not always audible. See the section on "Train Cars" for landmarks to aid in approaching the door area. Be careful not to get either cane or heel caught between the train and platform edge upon exiting.

Before exiting the train, it is sometimes possible to determine whether the platform is a side or a central platform by which door opens. Assuming that the rider is facing the direction in which the train is moving, if the doors open to the right the train is on a side platform; if they open to the left, it is on a central platform. The exception is at a split-level station or at the end of a line, where the train might pull into either track. Both doors can open at the National Airport station, where there are three tracks. See section on "Platforms." To locate the escalator to leave the platform level:

1. Follow the crowd.
2. Solicit aid.
3. Shoreline the platform edge, making sure the cane arc is sufficiently wide, until the escalator is audible.
4. Walk about 10 feet forward if on a central platform or to the barrier if on a side platform, and listen for auditory cues.

If unable to hear the escalator, walk parallel to the tracks until the escalator is audible. The rider may contact the metal railing under the back of the escalator, which can be followed to the front of the escalator. If contact is made with the cement wall or metal gate at the end of the platform, the rider should turn around and walk in the opposite direction.

Addfare Machine

When a farecard does not have adequate funds remaining to exit at the destination station, the farecard will be returned to the rider by the faregate without the barrier opening to allow exit.

The rider must upgrade the farecard at the addfare machine. There are two slots in the addfare machine located toward the left of the machine, one above the other. The lower slot is for inserting the original farecard. If no action is taken within a designated amount of time after inserting the farecard, the machine will return the card. The upgraded farecard is automatically released from the top slot after the required amount of money is inserted. Money is inserted in the bill and coin slots located to the right of the machine. The addfare machine will return the upgraded card when enough money has been inserted to allow the rider to exit at the faregate. The addfare machine cannot upgrade the farecard beyond this amount. It will automatically return any change forthcoming.

The blind rider does not need to know exactly how much money is required in order to exit, because the addfare machine will return any extra money deposited. Addfare machines are programmed to recognize the special senior citizen/handicapped farecards, and they will charge the appropriate reduced fare.

BAY AREA RAPID TRANSIT (BART) DISTRICT PLATFORM-EDGE DETECTION SYSTEM PROTOTYPE INSTALLATION AND MATERIALS EVALUATION

APPENDIX 2

Ralph S. Weule
Research by A.F. Peck and B.L. Bentzen,
Boston College

Section A

I. Installation

A. The platform-edge detection system was installed under contract 15NE 110 at Rockridge, Berkeley, and Montgomery Stations. This system consisted of installing raised strips on a 2-foot wide area along the entire platform edge. At each station, raised strips of PVC [polyvinyl chloride] material were used for one platform and raised strips of Epoxy Polyaggregate were used at the other platform. This installation was completed by February 20, 1985 at a cost of approximately $100,000.00 per station. (See Sections B and C for specifications.)

B. An additional type of detection material was found prior to the testing phase. A 100-foot section of this material, called tactile warning tile, was installed by the District at Lake Merritt Station. It is a rubber tile with raised bumps that alerts blind and visually impaired persons to the platform edge. This installation was completed on June 21, 1985, at a cost of $1,200.00 for materials only. (See Section D for specifications.)

C. The tactile warning tile described in paragraph B above was installed on the entire length of both platform edges at Lake Merritt Station. This installation was completed after the testing phase in January 1986 at a cost of approximately $25,000.00. (See Section D for specifications.)

II. Problems

A. In March of 1985, a slipping hazard was identified at Rockridge, Berkeley, and Montgomery Station platforms where the PVC raised ribs were installed. Immediate action was taken to apply a nonskid material to the surface of the raised ribs. This action eliminated the slipping hazard.

B. At Rockridge Station, platform two, an abnormal amount of water collects at low spots at a few locations on the platform. It is not known if this condition existed prior to installation of the raised ribs; however, maintenance is monitoring the problem to determine a possible fix.

III. Testing

A. Dr. Alec F. Peck and Ms. Billie Louise Bentzen of Boston College, under terms of an independent contract with the Urban Mass Transportation Administration, conducted formal tests of the platform-edge material installed at the four stations. Blind and visually impaired individuals, disabled people in motorized and nonmotorized wheelchairs, and disabled people with mobility problems took part in the tests. Bay Area Rapid Transit (BART) had no formal role in the design of these tests, which were completed in November 1985. (See Section E.)

B. Dr. Ian L. Bailey of the School of Optometry, University of California-Berkeley, evaluated the low vision aspects of the test materials, including color and contrast. This evaluation was completed in March of 1986.

C. BART maintenance personnel have reviewed the installations regarding wear and deterioration characteristics, cleaning and maintenance, water buildup, drainage, and ease of replacement. This evaluation was completed in April of 1986.

D. BART safety personnel have been tracking reports and comments received on the topic. The Safety Department has also videotaped the edges of Rockridge and Lake Merritt platforms in order to study the effects of the installation on all patrons, both handicapped and able-bodied. The number, type, and severity of incidents (falls, stumbles, etc.) arising at the four demonstration stations have been compared to the same data from other similar stations.

IV. Test Results

A. Boston College data analysis indicates that all of the installations were consistently detectable under the test conditions. Further, the tactile warning tile installed at Lake Merritt Station was statistically more detectable than the raised strip installations at Rockridge, Berkeley, and Montgomery Stations.

B. The low vision evaluation conducted by Dr. Ian Bailey, School of Optometry, University of California-Berkeley, indicates that the raised strips of PVC material and the tactile warning tile are satisfactory low vision stimuli. The raised strips of epoxy polyaggregate material do not provide a satisfactory contrast level to distinguish easily the strips from the platform materials.

C. BART maintenance evaluation of the test stations indicates the following:

1. No significant wear or deterioration is evident at any of the installations.

2. Cleaning is a problem at Rockridge, Berkeley, and Montgomery Stations. Dirt and debris collect between the raised ribs and cannot be machine cleaned. These areas have to be hand cleaned. The tactile warning tile at Lake Merritt Station is easier to clean.

3. Replacement or repair of damage to the edge strips at Rockridge, Berkeley, and Montgomery Stations would be difficult and labor-expensive due to the type of installation. The strips were glued into grooves cut into the platform edge. Replacement or repair would require considerable handwork, which would significantly increase the cost. Replacement of the tactile warning tile at Lake Merritt would be a relatively easy and inexpensive task. Worn or damaged 1-foot-square tiles can be easily replaced with no damage to the original surface.

4. Drainage and water buildup problems cannot be adequately evaluated at this time. Only one of the test stations (Rockridge) has outdoor platforms. Drainage problems at this station have been noted since the installation of the raised strips during periods of heavy rain. The 2-inch drainage gap should be adequate for the majority of outdoor stations. Problem areas will be taken care of on a case-by-case basis.

D. The Safety Department has been tracking reports for incidents associated with the test installations. A large number of incidents were noted immediately after the installation of the raised strips at Rockridge, Berkeley, and Montgomery Stations. These reports resulted from slips on the PVC material at the subject stations as stated above (see IIA.). After this hazard was eliminated in March 1985, there were no incidents or adverse comments submitted at the test stations. Further, during the test period (March 1985-March 1986) approximately 1.8 million patron crossings occurred at Rockridge Station,

5.35 million at Berkeley Station, and 10.5 million at Montgomery Station. A similar comparison of patron crossings at Lake Merritt Station is not possible due to the late installation of the tactile warning tile on the complete platforms (January 1986). However, during the 60-day test period at this station, approximately 280,000 patron crossings were recorded and no incidents or safety problems were noted.

V. Conclusion

The platform-edge detection system (tactile warning tile) installed at Lake Merritt Station is superior to the other materials installed at Rockridge, Berkeley, and Montgomery Stations.

A. Boston College independent test data analysis indicates that the tactile warning tile was statistically more detectable than the raised strip installations at Rockridge, Berkeley, and Montgomery Stations.

B. The low vision evaluation indicates that the tactile warning tile is a satisfactory low vision stimulus.

C. Tactile warning tiles are significantly less expensive to install, maintain, repair, or replace.

D. No safety-related incidents or adverse comments were noted since the installation of tactile warning tiles.

E. The synthetic rubber composition of tactile warning tile provides an additional benefit, as it provides insulation between the train and the platform. (This significantly reduces the car side touch potential associated with the traction power negative return.)

VI. Recommendation

That tactile warning tiles become the standard for platform-edge detection systems at BART and be installed at all station platforms.

Section B: Extruded Tactile Warning Strips

2.1 Materials.

2.1.1 Extruded tactile warning strips shall consist of an outdoor grade, ultraviolet stabilized polyvinyl chloride (PVC) rigid extrusion, conforming to ASTM Designation: D1784:13344-C.

2.1.1.1 The PVC extrusion shall have the following properties:

Property	Value	Test Method
Specific Gravity	1.46+0.02	ASTM D-792
Durometer "D"		
Hardness	82+3	ASTM D-785
Tensile Strength, psi	6,200	ASTM D-638
Tensile Modulus, psi	355,000	ASTM D-638
Flexural Strength, psi	11,300	ASTM D-790
Flexural Modulus, psi	410,000	ASTM D-790
Izod Impact (ft. lbs./inch)		
@ 77° F	3.80	ASTM D-256
Izod Impact (ft. lbs./inch)		
@ 32° F	1.78	ASTM D-256
Heat Distortion (F 264 psi)	163	ASTM D-648
Coefficient of		
linear expansion		
(inch/inch F x 10 -5)	3.3	ASTM D-696

2.1.1.2 The extrusion shall be black, and the color shall extend throughout the strip.

2.1.2 Epoxy adhesive shall be a solventless, rapid curing, stress relieved type, formulated primarily for use in bonding the tactile warning strip material to the grooved platform-edge material. Epoxy shall be furnished as two components, which shall be mixed together at the job site.

2.1.2.1 The epoxy adhesive shall have the following properties:

A. Properties of Cured Material (Cured 7 days @ 77°F—Tested @ 77° F)

Property	Value	Test Method
Tensile Strength, psi (MPa)	850 (5.8)	ASTM D-638

(continued)

Property	Value	Test Method
Tensile Elongation, %	85	ASTM D-638
Impact Resistance, in. lb. (J)	>160 (>18)	Gardner-Direct
Tensile Bond Strength to PCC, psi (MPa)	310 (2.1)	AASHTO T-237
Heat Deflection Temperature, F (C)	25 (−4)	ASTM D-648
Hardness Shore D	62	ASTM D-2240

B. Tensile Properties After Long Term Cure (ASTM D-628—3 mos. @ 77° F)

Property	Test Temperature		
	0°F (−18°C)	77°F (25°C)	140°F (60°C)
Ultimate Strength, psi	4,500 (31)	850 (5.8)	70 (0.5)
Tensile Elongation, %	7	85	10

Section C: Polyaggregate Epoxy Tactile Warning Strips

3.1 Materials.

3.1.1 Precast polyaggregate epoxy tactile warning strips shall consist of antislip filler securely bonded to a strip base. The strips shall be furnished in lengths of 10 feet 0 inch. The strip color shall be black and shall extend throughout the filler.

3.1.1.1 The antislip filler shall contain not less than 65% virgin grain aluminum oxide (A12O3) abrasive. The filler binder shall be a fully cured resilient type epoxy. The ratio of epoxy binder to filler shall be a minimum of 13%.

3.1.1.2 The strip base shall be extruded aluminum alloy 6063-T5.

3.1.1.3 Epoxy adhesive shall be a solventless, rapid-curing, stress-relieved type, formulated primarily for use in bonding the tactile warning strip insert material to the grooved platform edge material. Epoxy shall be furnished as two components, which shall be mixed together at the job site.

3.1.1.3.1 The epoxy adhesive shall have the following properties:

A. Properties of Cured Material (Cured 7 days @ 77°F—Tested 77°F)

Property	Value	Test Method
Tensile Strength, psi (MPa)	850 (5.8)	ASTM D-638
Tensile Elongation, %	85	ASTM D-638
Impact Resistance, in. lb. (J)	>160 (>18) 80 (9)	Gardner-Direct -Reverse
Tensile Bond Strength to PCC, psi (MPa)	310 (2.1)	AASHTO T-237
Heat Deflection Temperature, °F (C)	25 (−4)	ASTM D-648
Hardness Shore D	62	ASTM D-2240

B. Tensile Properties After Long Term Cure (ASTM D-638-3 mos. @ 77° F)

Property	Test Temperature		
	0°F (−18°C)	77°F (25°C)	140°F (60°C)
Ultimate Strength, psi (MPa)	4,500 (31)	850 (5.8)	70 (0.5)
Tensile Elongation, %	7	85	10

3.1.2 Cast-in-place polyaggregate epoxy tactile warning strips shall consist of antislip filler containing not less than 60% virgin grain aluminum oxide (A12O3) abrasive and a fully cured resilient-type epoxy binder. The ratio of epoxy binder to filler shall be a minimum of 13%. The strip of color shall be black and shall extend throughout the filler. The epoxy shall be furnished as two components, which shall be mixed together at the job site.

Section D: San Francisco BART District Specification for Platform-Edge Detection Tile October 18, 1985

I. Scope

The scope of this specification covers requirements that guarantee the essential doctrine of commonality and consistency of the platform-edge detection tile for the blind and the visually impaired pedestrian. *Form.* The platform-edge detection tile is in the form of a self-adhering synthetic rubber tile with a distinct pattern embossed on the surface.

Function. The function of the tile is to provide warning or direction by being detectable under foot and to provide a noticeably different sound when struck with the long cane, resulting in an audible input. Tile consists of a flat surface with tapered edges and with 41 raised truncated cones.

II. General Requirements

Material. The material shall be a synthetic rubber composition with the appropriate physical properties of resilience and high coefficient of friction. The material must also possess resistance to wear, weather, ozone, ultraviolet, and temperature to assure long life and durability in the proposed environment. The material must meet the following minimum standards.

Mechanical Properties.

Specific Gravity	0.97–0.99
Tensile Strength (ASTM D-412)	1100 psi
Ultimate Elongation (ASTM D-412)	350–400%
Hardness (Shore A)	70–75

Physical Properties.

1. The abrasion resistance as measured by the Tabar Test (ASTM D-3389) shows less than 0.63 gram weight loss.
2. The ozone resistance as measured by ASTM D518 shall exhibit no cracking after 70 hours at 50 pphm ozone concentration.
3. The weather resistance as measured by exposure for 1,000 hours shall exhibit little or no discoloration and less than 10% loss of tensile properties.
4. The temperature resistance as measured by ASTM D-746 shall exhibit a brittleness point of (minus) −55° F and long-term and long-term heat stability above 250° F.

Dimensions.

Width (mm)	300 mm
Length (mm)	300 mm
• Contour	DOT
• Overall Thickness (mm)	6.77
• Edge Thickness (mm)	1.00 mm

Surface Texture. Surface finish shall be a minimum of 60 rms and a maximum of 80 rms to increase coefficient of friction in wet and dry condition.

Color.

1. Yellow—Must conform to Federal Color No. 33538, as shown in Table V of Standard No. 595A.
2. Black—No. 37038.

III. Adhesive

The tile shall be supplied with a factory-applied pliant polymer adhesive with release paper. The adhesive must retain its back and adhesive qualities from −50° F to 140° F, and it shall meet the following requirements:

Thickness (Nominal)	0.032 Inches
Hardness (Shore A)	5-15
Solids	99%
Ash	40%
Elongation (77°)	500%
Force to Compress (ASTM C972)	80-165 lbs.
Flow (ASTM C639) (190° F)	0.020 (2 hrs.)
Yield Strength (ASTM C908) (77° F)	6 psi

Section E: Test Plan, BART Platform-Edge Warnings

A.F. Peck and B.L. Bentzen, Boston College (under contract with U.S. Department of Transportation, Transportation Systems Center, Cambridge, Massachusetts, DTRS57-84-P-81778, April 1985

The following plans present the tests to be conducted during the 1985 evaluation of the experimental edge warnings that have been installed for visually impaired travelers in selected BART stations. The plans have been designed to test (a) the detectability of the warnings underfoot, and T(b) the degree (if any) of difficulty which the warnings introduce for travelers who use wheelchairs.

Subjects

The pool of 30 subjects will be constructed in accordance with the following strata:

Age	N	Aid Type	N
5–21	5	dog	8–12
22–54	25	cane	18–22
55 and over	5		

The visual status of all subjects will be "totally blind," which will be defined as having remaining vision capability of no more than light perception. All subjects will be paid volunteers, each receiving an honorarium of $15.

Test Sites and Preparation

Three BART stations that have been outfitted with the experimental edge warning material will be used: Rockridge (R), Montgomery (M), and Berkeley (B). Each platform edge in the stations will be prepared in the following manner. At a point along the platform judged to be free of obstructions, the experimenter will draw three chalk lines: A. One line, 30 feet long, which intersects the platform edge at a 35-degree angle, with cross markings at 10, 20, and 30 feet. B. One line, 50 feet long, which intersects the platform edge at a 10-degree angle, with cross markings at 30, 40, and 50 feet. C. One line 20 feet long, which intersects the platform edge at a 90-degree angle, with cross markings at 7, 14, and 20 feet.

Order of Trials

The experimenter will be given a scoring sheet for each subject, on which the order of presentation of trials and the nature of each trial will be prescribed.

These predetermined trials will be organized in such a way that (1) each subject will perform two of the sighted guide trials in each of three stations, (2) each subject will perform two sighted guide trials at each of the three angles, and (3) each of the cane users will perform at both the 90-degree and 35-degree angles of approach on each of the platform edges in one station.

Dependent Measures

For both sighted guide and cane trials, the dependent measures will be (1) distance from platform edge to closest portion of subject's shoe and (2) number of steps taken on the tactile warning surface before acknowledgment of contact.

Procedure

Subjects will be familiarized with the warning strips in the following manner. The experimenter will take the subject to a position near the warning strip and will ask the subject to walk on and be aware of the texture of the platform underfoot. The experimenter will then ask the subject to place one foot to the left or right so that it will be on the warning strip, and will ask the subject if he or she can detect the difference between the two textures. The subject will be encouraged to move onto and off the textured edge warning until he or she believes that he or she can detect difference between the surfaces. The subject will then be instructed as follows: "I am going to guide you toward the warning material that you just felt. When you feel that warning again, I'd like you to stop immediately and tell me that you feel it underfoot. Remember to stop as soon as you feel the material underfoot. Any questions?" Each subject will then perform a total of six trials, using only a sighted guide. In addition, long cane users will perform four more trials, using their canes alone.

Sighted Guide Trials. Following a predetermined, counterbalanced order, the experimenter (sighted guide) will move the subject into position at one of the cross markings along one of the chalk lines. When the subject is comfortably in position, the experimenter will begin to walk at a normal pace along the chalk line, toward the platform edge. In the event that the subject does not recognize the warning material underfoot, the experimenter will continue to walk right up to the barrier at the edge of the platform.

Cane Trials. The subject will once again be moved to a position that was predetermined and will be told to "use whatever cane technique you would normally use in a BART station" and to stop when the edge warning material is detected.

Wheelchair Users Testing Plan. A group of 10 persons who travel using wheelchairs will be tested on six tasks involving the manipulation of wheelchairs on the edge-detection system to determine what effects the system may have on wheelchair travel. All tests will be performed on the epoxy-grit prototype. Results should be generalizable to other materials, such as coated PVC, having similar dimensions and friction characteristics. All tests will be conducted in Berkeley Station, which has a polished terrazzo floor adjoining the edge- detection system. Accor-

ding to the Advisory Committee, it is anticipated that of the three flooring materials in the three stations in which prototype warnings have been installed (Montgomery-brick; Rockridge-cement; Berkeley-terrazzo), wheelchair users are most likely to experience difficulties where the floor is smoothest, i.e., Berkeley. Therefore, the test will use the "worst case" situation.

All wheelchair participants will be asked to complete all six tasks. Participants will start from a location either on or near the edge-detection system and they will then move either across the system and onto or off of a vehicle or return to the main platform flooring (terrazzo). As each task is performed, the experimenter will collect the data, "Subject able to perform" or "Subject not able to perform." Following performance of the six tasks, participants will subjectively evaluate the effect of the edge-detection system on their use of BART. They will also give suggestions for techniques or strategies for minimizing these effects.

LIGHT RAPID AND LIGHT RAIL TRANSIT (LRT) LESSON PLANNING AID

APPENDIX 3

Dave Manzer
Kathryn Chew

The light rapid transit or light rail transit (LRT) lesson planning aid is a checklist for individualizing LRT system analyses and mobility lesson designs for students. It allows the instructor to review which skills and techniques should be included when providing instruction for students, be they rote or conventional travelers, and to record specific notes relevant to individual students, lessons, and transit system features. The checklist is a model whose items can be adapted for transit systems other than those found in Western Canada. (Some of the items below are explained further in "Light Rapid and Light Rail Systems in Western Canada.")

LRT Lesson Planning Aid

Factors to Consider	Comments
I. System design	
A. Complexity	
– Single line	
– Y, h, or x line	
B. Integration with conventional transit	
– Obstacles when transferring	
– Bus loop layout (for the bus loops that are integrated with LRT stations)	
II. Station design	
A. Modular/unique (route design can take into account complexity of stations)	
– Patterns	
– Location of access to street/platform	
– Train direction	

Factors to Consider	Comments
B. Lighting	
– Glare	
– High-contrast colors	
– Natural light	
– Artificial light	
C. Obstacles	
– Straight, unobstructed	
– Signage	
D. Security	
– Alcove and blind spots	
– Monitoring	
– Staffing	
E. Other	
III. Platform design	
A. Access	
– Number	
– Type (elevator, escalator, etc.)	
B. Platform-edge tactile/visual warning strip	
– Effectiveness	
– Size, location, textural differences	
C. Obstacles	
D. Other	
IV. Car design	
A. Exterior door buttons	
– Location	
– Ease of finding	
– Decal	
– Raised	
– Layout(s)	
B. Open doorway	
– Obstructed/unobstructed	
– Ratio of space between cars to space between doorjambs	
C. Interior door buttons	
– "Smart" door buttons	

(continued on next page)

Factors to Consider	Comments
– Side specific	
D. Seating	
– Special seating provisions	
E. Obstructions and handholds	
– Location	
– Hazards	
F. Other	
– Location of intercom	
– Station identification procedures	
V. Assistance available	
A. Staffing	
– Driver accessible for assistance	
– Conductor	
– Platform attendant	
– RTA (Rapid Transit Assistant)	
– Security staff	
B. Fare collection	
– Special pass	
– Type of regular fare collection	
– Proof of payment	

Factors to Consider	Comments
– Automated	
– Automated with attendant monitoring	
C. Public assistance	
– Pedestrian frequency	
– Multicultural ridership	
– Question-asking skills	
VI. Other considerations	
A. Platform recovery	
– Live rail location	
– Platform-solid/overhang	
– Separation from other hazards	
– Time/visibility to driver	
– Reliability of track intrusion system	
B. Staff training	
C. Information sharing	
D. Maps and memory aids	
– Auditory	
– Tactile	
– Visual	
VII. Preinstruction advocacy	

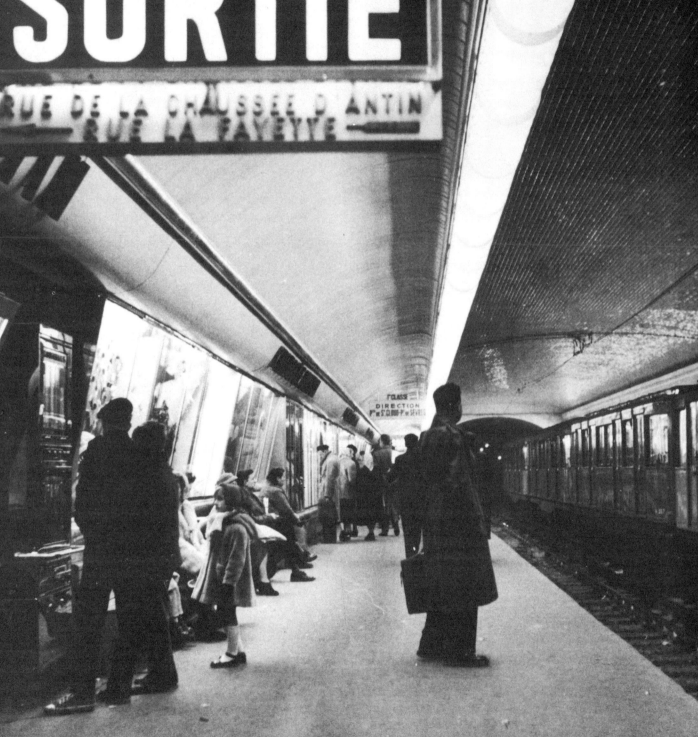

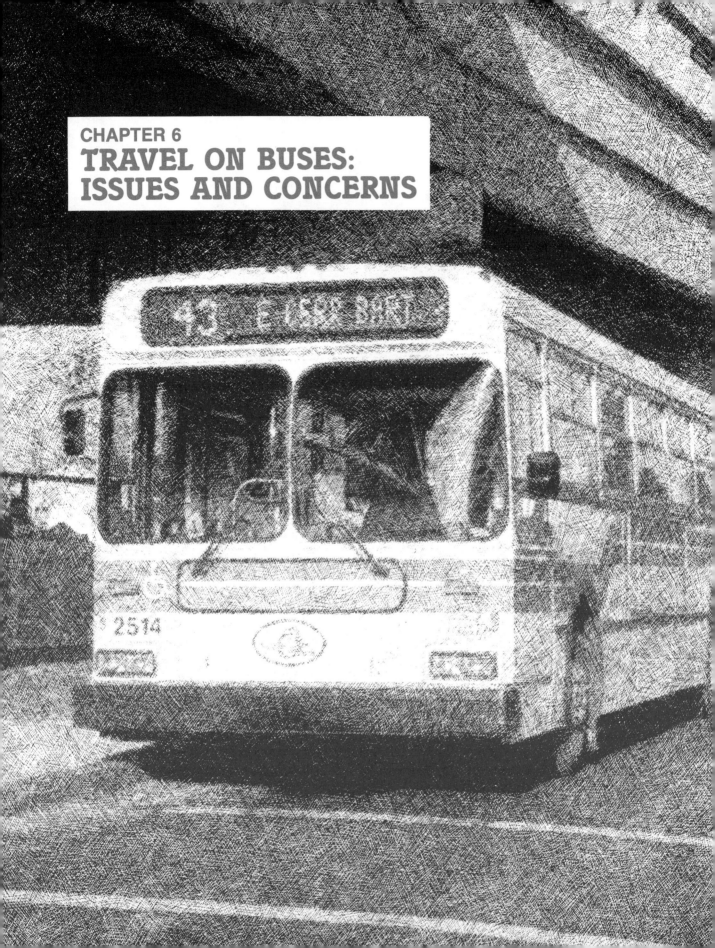

CHAPTER 6
TRAVEL ON BUSES:
ISSUES AND CONCERNS

Advocating in Behalf of Blind and Visually Impaired Bus Travelers

Toni Provost-Hatlen
Linda Alexander Myers

Bus travel today presents many difficulties for blind and visually impaired persons. But in many communities, precise and focused advocacy efforts are effecting change. Orientation and mobility (O&M) specialists in many different areas are accepting advocacy as a crucial aspect of their role and believe that their efforts have made a significant difference.

O&M specialists are not only teaching their students to travel independently, but they are also teaching them to advocate for themselves. Together, instructors and students must enlist mass transit officials and community agencies for blind and visually impaired persons in a joint venture to improve conditions for travelers with special needs.

Joining advisory committees on accessibility for local transit companies is one way to bring about change. These committees include members of various segments of the elderly and disabled population. It is important that blind and visually impaired people be represented at these advisory meetings in order to ensure that their needs and concerns will be addressed.

Improved accessibility is a goal of such committees. They are just as likely to provide technical advice on design and operations of transit projects as they are to provide ongoing reviews of policies that affect their constituencies. Their advise-and-consent role enables them to offer a wide range of consultation on topics including appropriate signage, the importance of accurate scheduling information, the need to educate drivers about various issues, and the development of new products that might assist blind and visually impaired riders.

Advocates need to present to mass transit authorities a list of particulars identifying problems and recommended solutions regarding blind and visually impaired passengers. The following examples illustrate the concerns and recommendations that were brought to the attention of a transit company in the San Francisco Bay Area by elderly and handicapped members of its advisory committee.

Improving Signage

Digital destination and route signs (called headsigns on buses) can be a challenge to read, not only for visually impaired persons but also for the general public. The difficulty of reading them became an issue only in recent years, when the traditional form of signs (called ''curtain'' signs) were replaced by electronic signs made up of luminous dots that can get dirty, fade, or malfunction. Although the legibility of the older signs is vastly superior to that of small-print electronic signs, transit companies prefer the latter because they have greater storage capacity for messages and are cost-effective. The recommendation of the advisory committee in San Francisco was to place a high-contrast, large-print bus number sign in the front windows of buses. The advisory committee members also requested that they be a part of the decision-making process when new headsigns were to be purchased. As a result of the committee's input, the transit company is presently purchasing large-print electronic signs that are much easier for all passengers to read. Some other recommendations of the advisory group include installing interior and exterior speakers on buses for announcing route information, providing large-print or brailled route schedules, enlarging the print size of bus numbers and destinations on bus pole signs, and designating bus poles with some sort of distinguishing feature that can be tactiley identified by blind people.

Promoting Accurate Information

Another problem that advocates can attempt to help solve is the inaccurate and misleading information given by some transit telephone operators answering calls from blind and visually impaired patrons. Misinformation clearly results in orientation and scheduling problems for the prospective traveler. The San Francisco advisory committee requested and received permission to observe the information operators on the job to get acquainted with their

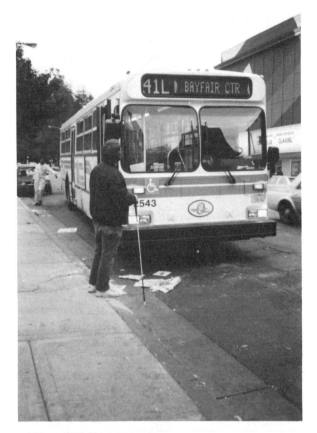

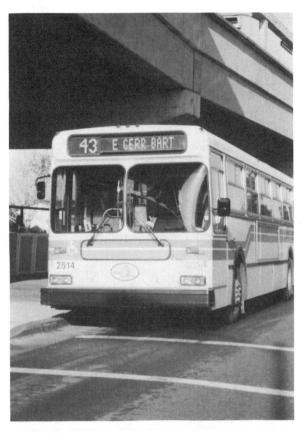

Because many people with low vision find it difficult to read the digital destination and route signs that have been installed in some bus systems, high-contrast, large-print bus number signs are often placed in the front windows of buses.

materials and procedures for giving information to callers. As a result of this visit, arrangements were made by members of the advisory committee to provide an in-service training program for the operators. One of the sessions took place at the Living Skills Center for the Visually Handicapped in San Pablo in order to give transit-information operators the opportunity to meet with blind and visually impaired riders and hear firsthand what a profound effect inaccurate information has on their ability to travel. The operators were also provided with the detailed information that blind and visually impaired callers need. As a result of these training sessions, information given by the operators has improved. Refresher training sessions will also be held periodically.

Advocating Training for Drivers

One of the most common problems in bus travel is that bus drivers lack an understanding of the needs of blind and visually impaired passengers. In an attempt to address this issue, the advisory committee provided sensitivity training concerning disabilities to all currently employed drivers. This experience demonstrated that sensitivity training sessions are most effective if they are compulsory and involve all transit personnel, including management. In addition to arranging for these training sessions, members of the advisory committee representing visually impaired passengers met with the head of the training department to learn what was included in the driver-training program regarding blind passengers. This meeting provided an opportunity to discuss the discrepancies between what drivers were being taught and what was, in reality, being practiced. The committee members also presented to the head of the training department a list of recommended ideas to be included in all future training programs. (See "Tips for Bus Drivers Dealing with Blind and Visually Impaired Passengers.") The advisory committee will continue to consult with the training department to improve drivers' awareness of the needs of blind and visually impaired passengers.

Using a Blueprint for Action

Advisory committees are an effective means of exploring and solving accessibility problems.

However, many other courses of action offer the possibility of effecting improvement. The following discussion outlines some specific suggestions for those who wish to influence transit authorities to implement changes in behalf of blind and visually impaired travelers. Travelers themselves and their families, rehabilitation agency staff, O&M specialists, and community activists all can adapt these action-oriented ideas to their own needs.

- Once an accessibility problem has been identified, call the transit company to let them know of your concern or complaint. Then document your request for action in a follow-up letter, and be sure to keep a copy for your own files. Transit

---

Tips for Bus Drivers Dealing with Blind and Visually Impaired Passengers

- It is helpful to tell a blind or visually impaired person the bus number and direction or final destination of the bus before he or she boards. Also, specify if it is an express bus.
- If you wish to direct a blind or visually impaired person to a seat, the seat adjacent to the door is preferable to the one behind you. A blind person will be more visible there, which will serve as a reminder for you to call out his or her stop.
- When handing a transfer to a blind or visually impaired person, place it directly in his or her hand rather than holding it out.
- It is very helpful to call out major cross streets so that a blind or visually impaired person can anticipate his or her stop.
- It is crucial to remember to call out a blind or visually impaired person's requested stop. It can be very disorienting if one is let off at an unfamiliar stop.
- If one driver relieves another, the first driver should be sure to inform the new driver to call out a blind or visually impaired person's desired destination.
- If at all possible, let a blind or visually

impaired person exit the bus in a spot free of poles, newspaper stands, etc. Otherwise, tell him or her that there are obstacles in front of the door.
- It can be helpful if the driver informs a blind or visually impaired person that he or she is exiting the bus at the curb or in the street a few steps away from the curb.
- Always let a blind or visually impaired person off at the bus stop. Otherwise he or she could become disoriented if let off someplace nearby but unfamiliar. If it is necessary to let the person off elsewhere, tell the person where you are letting him or her off.
- When giving directions to a blind or visually impaired person, use specific terms, such as "turn right or left" or "turn toward the front (or back) of the bus," rather than more general terms, such as, "over there" or "go that way."
- When a blind or visually impaired person exits the bus, it is helpful to tell him or her what street the bus is traveling on and whether the bus stop is on the near or far side of the cross street.

SOURCE: Living Skills Center for the Visually Handicapped, San Pablo, California.

One Woman's Campaign for Better Bus Signs

Wilma Seelye, an orientation and mobility (O&M) specialist in a big-city public school system, began to prepare to teach her visually impaired sixth-grade students local bus stop signs. Her problems immediately became apparent: How could she teach so many different signs and types, especially to such young students? Was there a purpose to all the variations? Soon, Seelye became a one-person activist in Michigan, asking for change and improvement to produce the kind of bus signs that would enable blind and visually impaired persons to travel with more confidence.

Blind and visually impaired people of all ages want to verify that they are, in fact, standing at a bus stop. Although drivers are required to pick up passengers holding a cane even if they are not standing exactly at the bus sign, they cannot be expected to know if someone without a cane is blind or visually impaired. In addition, it would be helpful for visually impaired travelers who use a telescope if the colors defining bus stops corresponded with the colors of the buses that stop there. Unfortunately, this is not always the case.

Wilma Seelye first contacted the local Office of Transportation, which refused to believe that 12 different styles of signs caused anyone a problem; the office was therefore reluctant to make any change. Then a local councilwoman was called, who immediately championed the cause for standardized, pictorial, color-coordinated bus stop indicators. The result? New pictorial signs were instituted with a visibility rating four times higher than that of the printed ones. These signs were designated for installation at every bus stop throughout the metropolitan area.

Pictorial signs benefit a large segment of the riding population, including visually impaired travelers, illiterate and mentally retarded citizens, and non-English-speaking passengers. "Our city's bus travelers now have signs visible to all," says this successful advocate.

—*Mark M. Uslan*

---

companies often look at the number of complaints registered or accidents reported when making decisions regarding future policies.

- If your transit company has an advisory committee dealing with the needs of disabled passengers, be sure to request that your concern is put on the agenda of their next meeting. Even if you are not a member of the committee, it is worthwhile to present your recommendations to them in person.

- In your files, document every telephone conversation, meeting attended, and commitment made by a representative of the transit company, noting the date it occurred (including the year) and the content of the discussion. Often, so much time passes between the original contact and the resolution of the problem that you will be glad to have your notes for reference.

- Follow-up is essential. Because blind and visually impaired people make up a small percentage of the total ridership of transit systems, requests and recommendations regarding visually impaired passengers are not always given top priority. Therefore, it is necessary to monitor the status of your recommendation continually to ensure that efforts are being made to address the matter. Be persistent if you want to get a response.

- If you do not receive a response in a reasonable amount of time, send a letter reminding the person with whom you are dealing of your request or recommendation, and send a copy to the person's supervisor or general manager. This procedure usually produces action.

- If all else fails, you may find it necessary to make a presentation directly to the board of directors involved. Board meetings are open to the public, and visitors are welcome to provide input. At these board meetings, decisions are sometimes made that have an impact on blind and visually impaired travelers. Ask that board meeting agendas be mailed to you in advance so that you can decide if you should attend. It is easier to prevent a problem before it starts than it is to remedy one already in existence.

- Involve the media when appropriate. Call television and radio stations and newspapers to bring attention to a matter of special concern to your community. The media can be used to reinforce any positive steps that a transit system is taking in regard to accessibility, and they can also be used to enlighten the public about an existing problem. Transit companies are concerned about their public image.
- If these approaches have proved unsuccessful in persuading a transit company to make reasonable accommodations for blind and visually impaired passengers, you may want to explore your legal options.

Many advocates have used such basic guidelines to improve travel for blind and visually impaired mass transit riders. (See ''One Woman's Campaign for Better Bus Signs.'') Advocacy alerts bus companies to the needs of the blind and visually impaired population and helps them make their systems responsive. It is an effective tool for creating change.

In-Service Training for Bus Drivers

Mark M. Uslan

When blind and visually impaired persons have to deal with unpredictable bus service and bus drivers who do not understand their needs, difficulties arise for them and the orientation and mobility (O&M) specialists helping them to increase their independence. In-service training has the goal of teaching drivers the important role they play in facilitating travel for blind and visually impaired passengers. Bus drivers need to learn to inform passengers of the bus number when the bus doors open at a bus stop, to call out major cross streets and transfer points, to remember to call out a blind or visually impaired passenger's requested stop, and to suggest that blind or visually impaired persons sit next to the door so they will not forget to call out requested stops. Training should also cover definitions of eye deterioration and diseases, explanations of the particular problems of deaf-blind travelers, and the needs of other people with special conditions or disabilities, such as epilepsy or mental retardation.

Videotapes for Training

The use of a movie or videotape in training sessions is useful in relaxing participants and creating a comfortable and informal atmosphere. Most important, videotapes in driver education programs can heighten the sensitivity of drivers to the needs of blind and visually impaired and multidisabled riders. They can show and explain a variety of disabilities. In one case, special filters were used in filming to simulate different visual impairments. Videos can use several locations and different riders to replicate situations that occur in everyday bus travel for blind and visually impaired passengers. In addition, interviews with these riders, relating how they deal with their impairments on a day-to-day basis and how they rely on the transit system to maintain their independence, can highlight their goals and their needs much more graphically than any lecture can.

In Broward County, Florida, a transit safety and training official approached the state's Division of Blind Services and requested help in producing in-service training sessions for all new bus operators (Hanley, 1986). The first five training sessions were conducted at bus terminal classrooms. Each class was shown a movie entitled *What Do You Do When You Meet a Blind Person?* (American Foundation for the Blind, 1971) followed by a question-and-answer period. A videotape entitled *Blind Awareness Training Session for Mass Transit Bus Operators* (1986) has also emerged from the Broward County experience. This videotape contains information and sta-

New Products: Helping the Driver and the Passenger

Bus identifiers are currently being used to determine the bus needed by visually impaired or deaf-blind riders in multibus zones in Seattle, Washington. These travelers carry and display specially designed route number cards, giving bus drivers a quick and effective way of identifying a disabled passenger.

The cards for visually impaired persons have black numbers on a white background; for deaf-blind riders the black numbers are on a yellow background. They are packaged in a clear plastic holder with extra pockets for spare numbers, the rider's bus pass, and a taxi card as well. Riders display the bus route that they want.

A special-assistance green destination card printed in large-size type gives the bus route number, the bus stop where the traveler gets on the bus, and the desired destination on one side and return route information on the other. This card is handed to the driver when the rider boards the bus. If the rider is on the correct bus, the driver places the card on the transfer clip or clipboard and helps seat the passenger in the courtesy section if that assistance is needed. The driver calls out the desired destination stop and returns the card when the passenger leaves, again offering assistance if necessary. Should the rider board the wrong bus, the driver immediately returns the card, indicating the mistake.

—*Gloria M. Sanborn*

tistics about blind and visually impaired travelers, how they can be identified, how they are taught to travel independently, some of the problems they encounter, what bus operators can do to help, and directions for a blindfold experience.

In Seattle, Washington, a 20-minute driver education videotape is currently training 1,100 full-time drivers and 900 part-time drivers who operate over 1,000 coaches. This video focuses on communicating with blind, visually impaired, and deaf-blind riders, calling out bus stops, and becoming aware of the needs of dog guide users. It stresses the importance of drivers' scanning the front of the bus zone before pulling out into the street and the use of exterior speakers (which are not available in every system) to announce route numbers. It also indoctrinates drivers in the use of newly developed bus identifiers and special-assistance cards. (See "New Products: Helping the Driver and the Passenger.") For the benefit of all passengers, the video emphasizes courtesy, consideration, patience, and respect.

Many training programs use a blindfold experience as an additional teaching device. Each bus operator chooses a partner for what is called a trust walk. In this exercise, one person is blindfolded and holds the arm of the guide, and then the roles are reversed. Afterward, feelings about this experience are explored, and final questions can be asked.

Communication Between Transit Personnel and Passengers

Communication between bus drivers and their passengers is an effective way to stimulate drivers' interest in and sensitivity toward passengers' needs. Blind and visually impaired travelers can share their frustrations, experiences, and suggestions with drivers. This interaction can help drivers meet the needs of the blind and visually impaired community. A field trip to an agency or center for blind and visually impaired people can allow bus drivers to observe the skills that are taught and demonstrate to them how blind and visually impaired people can function independently.

Group seminars are another useful device in improving communication. Seminars conducted by O&M specialists can bring together representatives of the local transit authority and blind and visually impaired people to allow a free-flowing exchange

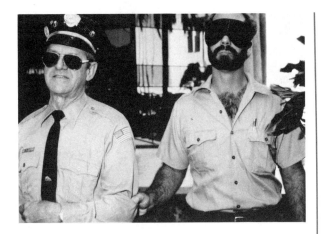

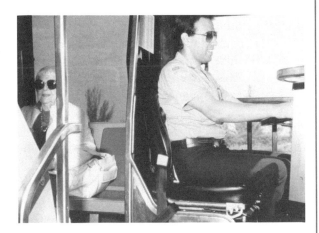

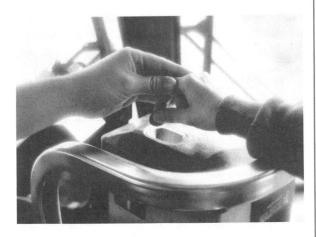

Bus drivers who have participated in training programs understand the challenges faced by blind and visually impaired travelers and know the specific forms of help that they need.

of information and, as important, feelings. Having staff psychologists in attendance facilitates these open discussions, which, over time, can result not only in improved communication but also in positive and effective problem solving.

These kinds of training activities and interactions improve the quality of services for blind and visually impaired travelers and create a positive and cooperative working relationship between local transit authorities and the blind and visually impaired community. Certainly the latter must exert every effort to help transit companies provide this kind of training, especially when they lack the resources or personnel to proceed on their own. When drivers understand the courage shown by a blind or visually impaired person who travels independently, they are bound to exhibit more empathy and willingness to help.

ELSIE, the Talking Bus Stop in England

Ann Frye

"It enables us to keep our independence" was the comment of one blind passenger about the experimental talking bus stop system being used in the west of England. ELSIE, as the Electronic Speech Information Equipment is known, was conceived and designed with exactly this aim in mind. The idea of ELSIE was first proposed to the Department of Transport in London by Dr. Tony Heyes of the Blind Mobility Research Unit at Nottingham University as part of a process of looking at ways in which modern technology could be harnessed to alleviate some of the mobility problems experienced by blind and visually impaired people.

Like all other developments undertaken before and since by the department concerning mobility for disabled people, the project was devised in consultation with organizations representing blind and visually impaired people. Their comments and advice were sought and attended to at every stage of its development.

Components of the System

The problems confronting many blind and visually impaired people who have to rely on public transportation are similar everywhere: They have considerable difficulty in locating bus stops, establishing whether the bus they need stops at a given stop, discovering when the next bus is scheduled to arrive, and, finally, ascertaining which approaching bus is the one they need. A sighted person can obtain all this information from visual observation or by reading the timetables posted at bus stops, but a blind or visually impaired person must seek the assistance of a sighted passerby—if there happens to be one in the vicinity.

Given the problems encountered by blind and visually impaired bus passengers, the project's objective was to devise a system that would enable a blind or visually impaired person to locate a bus stop and manually activate some audible information about the bus service provided at the stop, scheduled arrival times, and the approach of any given bus. The system that was developed revolved around three main components: a "talking" element that used voice synthesis, a bus identification unit that "read" the route numbers of approaching buses, and, linking these two components, a coordinating system that used a microcomputer.

Use of Voice Synthesis

For the talking element of the system, it was essential to use voice synthesis rather than a tape recording. It was decided that ELSIE had to be able to speak over 10,000 unique phrases. In a system in which continuous speech is assembled from a library of phrases, it must be possible to select each phrase at exactly the right moment and not be forced to wait for a part of a phrase. If all the separate phrases are on a recorded tape, there inevitably are long gaps while the tape rewinds to the right place. The voice synthesis process employed for an application like ELSIE, in which high-quality speech is necessary, makes use of a technique that allows words or complete phrases to be encoded.

To make the synthesizer, each word or phrase is spoken into a machine that analyzes the sound and allocates a whole string of codes to each sound. This coding process even takes into account the pitch and quality of speech. For instance, a female voice produces a different set of code numbers from a male voice. These codes are then stored in the synthesizer in very fast-operating memory units, similar to those used in a computer. When a phrase is to be uttered by the synthesizer, the codes are fed rapidly into the unit, and sound signals equivalent to those codes are regenerated and emerge as speech. This process happens so quickly that it is possible to jump sequentially from one coded word to the next and thus to string together all the words needed to make a whole sentence.

Identification of Buses

Another component of the system involves detecting and identifying the route numbers of approaching buses. This can be done technically in a number of ways. For example, a television camera can be pointed toward the bus approach path, and pictures from the camera can be fed into a small roadside microcomputer that is able to analyze all the elements of the image and identify the route number shown on the destination board of an approaching bus. This technique is promising but is likely to be expensive. Another system under development utilizes a concept similar to that used in a television set's remote control. In this system, a small infrared-light transmitter is mounted on top of the bus and continuously emits the code of the bus's route number. An infrared receiver at the bus stop detects and decodes the emitted bus signals.

The technique used in the initial trials of the talking bus stop involves a small, low-power radio transmitter mounted by the road, approximately 200 yards ahead of the bus stop. An aerial loop is buried just beneath the road surface and radiates a radio signal picked up by a small receiver carried beneath each bus. When a bus's receiver recognizes the calling signal, it responds by transmitting another radio signal back into the road loop. This return signal carries coded information that the equipment on the road can translate into the bus's route number. The route number can be set by simple switches in the driver's cab.

To link together the voice synthesis equipment with the bus detection equipment, a microcomputer comes into play. The computer also holds information about the current date, holidays, weekends, events, time of day, and current timetable information for all buses.

Operation of the System

A simplified schematic diagram of all the elements of the system is shown in Figure 1. The system consists of a small box mounted on the bus stop post or within the bus shelter. This box houses the loudspeaker from which the synthesized speech will emanate and a push button that, when operated, initiates an announcement of bus number and timetable information. To help blind and visually impaired people locate the box, the unit emits a continuous audible clicking sound at the rate of about one click per second. When the button is pressed, the announcement is made in the following form: "Good morning. The time is 10:23 a.m. Buses using this stop are: The number one-0-four; next bus due at 11:25; the number one-0-five; next bus due at 10:30. I will tell you which bus is approaching." The time of day spoken is the actual time to the nearest minute. The announcement is for the scheduled time of arrival for the next bus for each route using the stop.

Whenever a route and time announcement is requested, the unit becomes ready to identify approaching buses. If no requests are made, the equipment remains silent, aside from emitting its continuous clicking sound. When the equipment is activated, each approaching bus is identified and the route number and destination are announced. Each announcement of an approaching bus is pre-

Figure 1. The primary elements of Electronic Speech Information Equipment (ELSIE).

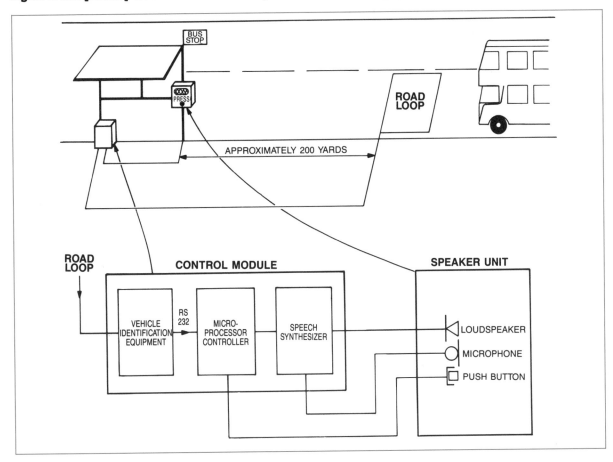

ceded by a two-tone sound signal that alerts waiting passengers to the imminence of an announcement. The system recognizes and announces all buses operating at a given stop until it has announced at least one bus for every route. It will then make no further announcements until the button is pressed again to obtain timetable information.

If the unit is in the middle of announcing route timetable information and an approaching bus is detected, the phrase being spoken will be completed and will be followed immediately by the announcement of the approaching bus's number. This will take the following form: "(Chime) The number one-0-five is approaching."

Noise Control

To make sure that ELSIE does not become a nuisance in quiet residential areas because of overloud or persistent announcements, the bus stop units have a built-in microphone that listens to the ambient noise of the street. The level of the noise is then used for controlling the volume of the announcement. That is, if the street noise is loud, the announcement will be spoken with a volume high enough to be heard by a listener close by. If the street noise is low—during the evening, for example—the sound level of the speech unit will be reduced accordingly. As a further measure to reduce the nuisance effect of the system, all announcements are stopped when the time of the last bus has passed. The equipment is then reactivated the following day just before the first bus is due.

In even the best-run systems, there are times when, for various reasons, the buses on some or all routes are either not running or are running irregularly. To allow for these situations, the equipment can make appropriate announcements. These messages are given in response to the push-button request for information, and at the same time the announcements of impending bus arrivals continue in the usual way.

Field Testing

The area chosen for the field trial of ELSIE was the small town of Weston-Super-Mare in the west of England, a seaside town with a population of 57,000. Although the town has a register of blind and visually impaired people totaling 300, there are many more people with impaired vision who, for one reason or another, are not on the register and more still who come to the town as holiday visitors. Like many other seaside resorts in that part of the country, Weston has a disproportionately large elderly population. The town also houses a residential hotel that caters specifically to blind and visually impaired visitors from London, which means that there is a constant stream of blind and visually impaired people who are unfamiliar with the town and who need to travel around via public transport.

For the field trial, nine bus stops in and around the town center were equipped, along with about 40 buses. Ordinarily, bus route numbers are set by the drivers prior to the start of their runs. To check that the correct settings were made, equipment installed in the bus garage read the code radiated by each bus and showed the route numbers on a large display unit.

The equipment performed technically well. There were, perhaps inevitably, a few adjustments necessary in the early days of the trial, in particular to the aerial road loop. One major concern—that the bus stop push-button units would be vandalized—proved to be unfounded. Nothing worse happened to the units than the appearance of some minor graffiti (although the boxes were deliberately made of a particularly impenetrable material).

In addition to checking the technical feasibility and reliability of the system, the main purpose of the trial was to see whether ELSIE was effective in helping blind and visually impaired people to travel independently. To find out passengers' responses to the system, a questionnaire was drawn up, which was widely circulated to both residents and visitors in the area. Produced in large print and in braille as well as in standard print, it was distributed by the local association of blind people.

The comments of users and participating organizations made it clear that the system was well received and extremely welcome. Its usefulness not only in helping blind and visually impaired people, but also in giving guidance and reassurance to elderly people and to visitors unfamiliar with the town's bus system and routes was demonstrated. One suggestion, already implemented, was to have ELSIE announce the destination of approaching buses as well as their route numbers. This information is particularly valuable for out-of-town visitors. Other suggestions under consideration include increasing the volume of announcements and incorporating into the system the ability to stop ELSIE once the required information has been given. The first might cause complaints among local residents, while the second may present technical difficulties.

ELSIE's benefits are not exclusively for bus passengers. It is possible to use the system for a variety of management purposes, including internal monitoring and traffic control. As with so many items of equipment or facilities for people with disabilities, the more general the application and the wider the advantages, the more likely companies or government agencies will be willing to make the necessary investment.

Although ELSIE is still just one experimental system operating in one small town in the west of England, it has the potential to become more widely adopted. Not only will it enable more blind and visually impaired people to use buses independently and to do so with more confidence and less anxiety, but it will also benefit other bus passengers, bus operators, and the bus industry as a whole.

How Japan Accommodates Its Bus Travelers

Sam C.S. Chen

Bus travel in Japan is as important as rapid rail travel is to both the sighted and the blind and visually impaired population. At the same time that innovations were being introduced in the subway and train systems in Tokyo to facilitate travel for blind and visually impaired riders (see "Some Solutions to Problems Encountered by Blind and Visually Impaired Travelers in Tokyo" in Chapter 5), similar

accommodations were being made in the bus system.

In recognition of the great difficulty that blind and visually impaired travelers may encounter in locating the right bus stop and boarding the correct bus, certain accommodations and adaptations have been made in Tokyo to overcome common problems. Some of these adaptations address both problems in bus travel and problems in traveling the streets of Tokyo. (See "Guides for Pedestrian Safety in Tokyo.") The following discussion describes some of the highlights of the improved system.

Audiotaped Messages

In order to provide blind travelers with accurate information in an efficient manner, a special device has been installed inside the railings of the stairs that lead to bus terminals. Since the terminals are often divided into different areas that are connected to different stairs, blind and visually impaired travelers may locate the right bus terminal via audiotaped messages that are activated when the top end of the railing is touched.

Braille Blocks

When a bus stop is near a crosswalk or intersection, brailled blocks [tiles] embedded in the sidewalk lead blind and visually impaired travelers from one end of the crosswalk directly to the bus stop. If the bus stop is located in the middle of the street block, the braille blocks are located beside and about 20 feet to either side of the bus stop. After a traveler finds a braille block, he or she may look for the signpost marking the bus stop.

A 2-foot-wide yellow square is located at each bus stop to indicate exactly where one can board a bus. The marker can be detected by foot or cane. The presence of this boarding spot makes it incumbent upon bus drivers to pull in at the same place each time. Drivers are instructed to position their buses so that a person standing on the square will be able to step into the bus when the door opens.

Bus Driver Training

Bus driver training goes beyond the positioning of the buses. Bus drivers always announce the route

Guides for Pedestrian Safety in Tokyo

In addition to Japan's rapid rail and bus service improvements, several safety precautions have been undertaken for blind travelers so that they can walk safely on the streets of Tokyo. The following are some of the highlights of these features:

- Shiny yellow blocks, which are easily detected by feet or cane, are located at the edge of the sidewalk. The braille blocks are also used to guide blind travelers from a train station or bus stop to a variety of facilities, such as City Hall, shopping malls, a braille library, the rehabilitation center, and a school for the blind.
- Auditory devices are often used in various places. In some areas, where the layout of the streets seems to be confusing, an auditory device that emits continuous signals is used to guide blind travelers. The post to which the device is attached serves as a landmark that blind and visually impaired pedestrians can use to reorient themselves. In addition, audio devices are often installed in the entrances to public buildings to guide blind and visually impaired persons.

- There are a number of different kinds of street intersections in Tokyo. Some are shaped as normal cross intersections, others are somewhat irregular, and in some places more than four streets intersect each other. It was deemed necessary, therefore, to install some type of guiding system to assist blind and visually impaired persons in crossing these streets safely and reaching their correct destinations. Audible traffic signals that emit pleasing music in a march tempo were accordingly installed beside the regular traffic signals on certain streets. These devices are electronically connected to the traffic light's circuit, and the music can be heard as long as the pedestrian cross stays green. Blind and visually impaired travelers are assured that the traffic has been stopped when they hear the music.

These advances have enabled blind and visually impaired travelers to walk the streets of Tokyo not only in greater safety but also with increased self-confidence. Accommodations such as those described are easily transferable to other cities and areas.

—*Sam C.S. Chen*

numbers and destinations of their buses to persons waiting to board at the bus stop. This audible message is essential for blind and visually impaired persons because buses traveling several different routes frequently share the same stop.

Concerned about the safety and ease with which blind and visually impaired persons use the bus system, Tokyo's transportation authorities want to be assured that these travelers are informed about routes and their present location at any time. Bus drivers, therefore, even inform passengers of road conditions, such as upcoming sharp turns or bumps that may cause them discomfort.

Other Accommodations

There are additional ways that travel has been made easier for blind and visually impaired bus riders in Tokyo:

- The bus fare machine is found at the entrance of the bus. Money is deposited in the box, and change is received at the bottom.
- Several seats on the bus are reserved for physically disabled passengers. The seats are located close to the entrance for easy access and safety. A sign over the seats clearly indicates that they are reserved for disabled persons. However, peo-

ple with disabilities are under no obligation to use these seats if they do not wish to do so.

- Immediately after a bus leaves a stop, an audio message, normally recorded on tape, informs passengers of upcoming stops. Prior to the next stop, another message announces the next stop and provides information about transfers and the public facilities near the stop, such as hospitals, libraries, and shopping malls. These messages are invaluable for blind and visually impaired passengers and help them avoid the delay and inconvenience of missed stops.

With over 11 million residents in Tokyo proper alone, the transportation systems are fully utilized and vital to the life of the city. Creative changes in mass transit, such as those described in the bus system, can only expand and enrich the lives of the members of the blind and visually impaired community. At the same time, benefits accrue to the sighted population as well. Orientation and mobility (O&M) specialists providing services in this environment have the support of the mass transit system itself, giving them greater opportunities for greater success among a wider group of clients.

References

American Foundation for the Blind (AFB). (1971). *What do you do when you meet a blind person?* [Film]. New York: Phoenix Films.

Broward County Division of Blind Services. (1986). *Blind awareness training session for mass transit bus operators.* [Film]. Florida: Broward County Division of Blind Services.

Hanley, D. (1986). Broward County mass transit: Meeting the needs of the blind and visually impaired. *Journal of Visual Impairment & Blindness,* **80**(1), 542-543.

PART III

ORIENTATION AND MOBILITY TRAINING: APPROACHES AND TECHNIQUES

BLIND AND visually impaired travelers who strive for increased and improved mobility are one variable in the mass transit equation explored in this book. Transit authorities and urban planners who pursue a better knowledge and understanding of the needs of blind and visually impaired passengers are another. The specialists responsible for providing blind and visually impaired persons with the experience and training for travel in mass transit are the third.

Training for travel in mass transit systems is part of the orientation and mobility (O&M) curriculum for blind and visually impaired persons. From coast to coast in the United States and in cities abroad, the complexities of mass transit in both rail and bus systems are acknowledged. But so is the broad range of techniques and strategies available to O&M specialists for dealing with these systems.

From the needs of young visually impaired children through those of students in secondary school and young people moving into adulthood, O&M training encompasses the particular requirements and abilities of the student, the role of family members, and the obligation of the specialist to create productive working relationships. When it comes to independent travel, building self-confidence goes hand in hand with assessing clients and understanding the transit system each must challenge. Nevertheless, one can view the different settings, features, and sizes of various rapid rail and bus systems and recognize the common thread running through them: The problems exist, but the solutions are workable.

In all cases, O&M specialists can approach problems in specific areas and find that they have general application. Instructional preparation and philosophy, sequenced training, both in the classroom and on site, and familiarization techniques all provide viable, practical plans for comprehensive orientation. As more blind and visually impaired persons are taught the skills and techniques needed for mass transit travel, O&M specialists who do their jobs will, by extension, effect change and improvement in the systems their clients use.

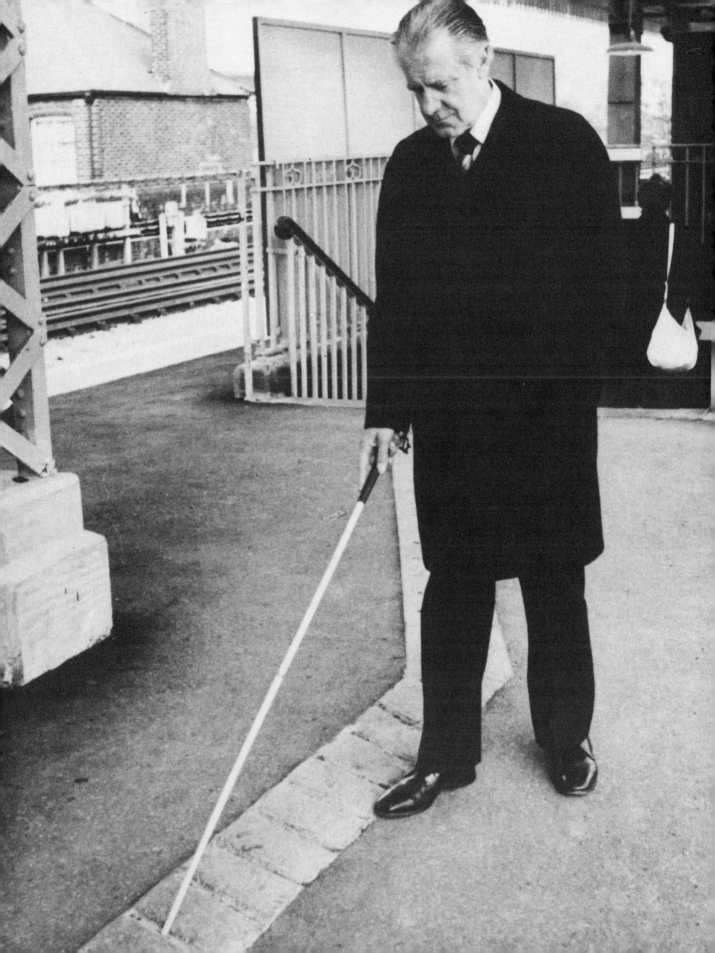

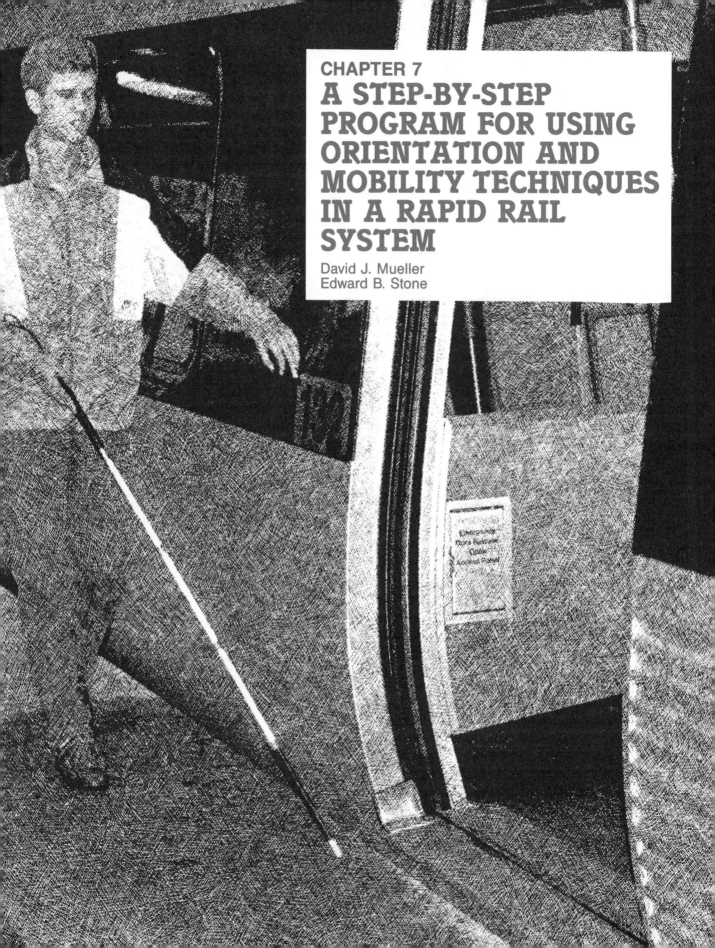

CHAPTER 7
A STEP-BY-STEP PROGRAM FOR USING ORIENTATION AND MOBILITY TECHNIQUES IN A RAPID RAIL SYSTEM

David J. Mueller
Edward B. Stone

In a large metropolitan city, rapid rail travel can be dangerous and confusing. One can easily understand the apprehension that affects many blind and visually impaired people when they contemplate using one of these systems with inadequate training. In recognition of these real dangers, a sequential plan of instructional procedures was developed to enable students in Atlanta, Georgia, to use rapid rail safely, efficiently, and independently.

The program that will be outlined here has been extremely successful in training students in the Atlanta area to use the Metropolitan Atlanta Rapid Transit Authority (MARTA) system. Given the variation in other systems, slight lesson changes may be necessary when the program is applied to other locations. But the basic orientation and mobility (O&M) procedures remain the same, and the teaching results should be similar. When students complete and master the O&M techniques provided in the program, they should be able to transfer some or all of their skills to travel in any other rapid rail system.

Guidelines for O&M Specialists

Taking all the variables into consideration, O&M specialists can begin training by creating a serious but relaxed atmosphere to help alleviate students' fears. They can proceed to follow basic guidelines that O&M specialists need to follow in preparing lessons. (See "Guidelines for Rapid Rail Training.") To begin, they must totally familiarize themselves with the transit system that will be used during training, and that includes getting to know both management as well as security personnel. These are the people with whom they must discuss various procedures. In addition, all initial training should be done at one station that does not experience much passenger activity. When a given student is ready, busier stations and stations with other designs may be introduced.

Before students can begin training on a rapid rail system, they should be able to demonstrate properly and proficiently these variations of standard cane techniques involving extensive contact with the ground surface: touch-and-slide, touch-and-drag, and the constant-contact method [see glossary for

definitions]. Students must be knowledgeable about the use of compass directions, the ability to identify

Guidelines for Rapid Rail Training

These simple guidelines can be followed in training blind and visually impaired people to use any rapid rail system:
1. Use compass directions.
2. Determine if there are similarities in station designs or the location of public conveyances within the system.
3. Find out if there are similarities in track locations in stations within the system. For example, in Atlanta's system, these principles can be followed:
   a. When in an east-west station on a single-track platform, turn south for the westbound train and north for the eastbound train.
   b. When in a north-south station on a single-track platform, turn east for the southbound train and west for the northbound train.
   c. When in an east-west station on a double-track platform, turn north for the westbound train and south for the eastbound train.
   d. When in a north-south station on a double-track platform, turn east for the northbound train and west for the southbound train.
4. Determine if there is a system or rationale behind the colors or appearance of lettering or signs. For example:
   a. Red signs might depict north-south trains.
   b. Blue signs might depict east-west trains.
   c. Signs with large print might depict double-track platforms.
   d. Signs with smaller print might depict single-track platforms.
5. Determine if a pattern exists in multiple-train stations with steps and escalators. For example:
   a. Steps go to single-track platforms only.
   b. Escalators go to double-track platforms only.

changes in textures and surfaces, the use of landmarks and clues, and the proper procedures for soliciting help from the public. Auditory alignment skills and as strong a sense of spatial imagery as possible are important for staying oriented to the location of the tracks and across open station areas. Students should master all the necessary orientation skills, process the information they have gathered, and be able to give this information to the instructor in an organized fashion. O&M specialists provide direct instruction when teaching specific cane techniques or helping students to extract important orientation information. They must assume the role of trainer, observer, and guardian.

Procedures

The training program developed in Atlanta involved phases in the classroom, in the transit station, and on the platform and train. The program is presented here in the form of instructions for O&M specialists.

In the Classroom

The first phase of instruction is performed in the classroom. Discuss the history, development, and operation of the transit system that will be used in the training, including how many miles the system encompasses, the number of stations, and the direction of the rail lines. Explain the operational details of the system, including the power source used to propel trains, how this power is transferred to trains, the location of the electrified, or "hot" rail, and the number of rails on which the trains ride. These details are interesting and educational, as well as necessary for training and safety.

Next, describe how the bus system connects to the rail system, the cost of fares, how to obtain a farecard, and how to use a transfer between the two systems. Provide basic diagrams of some stations and let students know where historical, civic, commercial, and entertainment facilities are located relative to specific stations. These facts provide both information and incentive.

The process of obtaining half-fare or discount cards for disabled and elderly passengers can be started in the classroom and then moved to one of the designated outlets where cards are sold. Students need to know that a physician's eye report, a social security card, and a personal identification card, complete with photograph and home address, are usually required. Explain all procedures, the times during the day when cards can be used, and the card expiration date. Role-play the process of getting a half-fare card until students feel comfortable enough to go to the actual facility and obtain a card independently.

The next lesson concerns the design of stations and passenger waiting areas. If necessary, use diagrams. Atlanta's rapid rail system, for example, has three basic station designs consisting of one to four levels above ground, below ground, and a combination of both. Each station may have from one to three types of passenger waiting areas: single-track platforms, double-track platforms, or a combination of the two. The differences among these three variations should be explained to students.

Later on, some students may become capable of identifying a station's design upon entering the station by using self-familiarization techniques and compass directional concepts. For instance, they may come to recognize that if stairs and escalators from the concourse level to platforms are not found along the station's perimeter, the centrally located ones will nearly always lead to double-track platforms. They may also learn that double-track platforms are to be expected at the ends of rail lines.

After becoming familiar with typical station designs and what can be expected from them, students may be able to use other lines more fully by applying in other stations what they learned in their initial instruction. They may also utilize their knowledge of compass directions to locate platforms.

In the Station

After classroom training, it is time to explore stations. The first outdoor lesson will take students to several stations to explore specific landmarks or architectural designs that can be associated with station entrances. In Atlanta, each station has a metal grate on the ground at the entrance and a large white

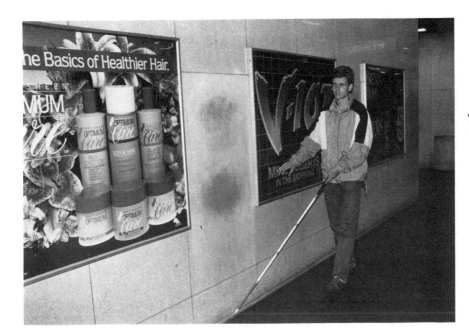

Trailing walls is a technique blind persons use to familiarize themselves with a station.

pole with three colored strips on it and the acronym "MARTA." After they have located these kinds of landmarks, students can listen for typical sounds from inside the station, such as escalators and train announcements. Once they cross a landmark, they should use a constant-contact cane technique and walk at a slower pace.

Inside the station, the task is to locate both the token machine and the turnstiles, using self-familiarization techniques. Assist students in identifying the various parts of each machine. Let them practice inserting a dollar bill by going through the following steps: (1) hold the bill lengthwise and insert it into the machine, (2) if the machine rejects the bill, remove it, turn it over lengthwise, left to right, and reinsert it into the machine, (3) should the machine reject it again, remove it, turn it over toward the machine, and reinsert. The bill should be accepted by the machine within four attempts.

After students receive a token or rail pass, auditory skills should be used to help locate and proceed to the turnstiles. Have students count the turnstiles, identify the turnstile for people with special needs and the sound it makes when someone exits incorrectly, locate any other important features or ac-

cessories on the turnstiles, such as an assistance telephone, and use the turnstiles.

Once through the turnstile, students must first employ systematic search patterns to become familiar with the area. They should be able to identify the ground texture inside the turnstile and any other texture changes encountered. During this self-familiarization process, have them point to the turnstiles from various locations. When this technique is accomplished, they should be able to describe, by using compass directions, the location of the turnstiles, the turnstile for disabled people (if there is one), the assistance telephone, the public telephones, steps, elevators, escalators, and exits. As part of this lesson, students can practice using the assistance telephone to solicit information about train arrivals and departures and track locations.

On the Platform
Proceed to the train level where the students will become familiar with the platform edge and the tactile warning strip, if there is one. To become familiar with the tactile warning strip, students should identify the texture first with the cane and then with their hands. Next, have them turn in the direction of the

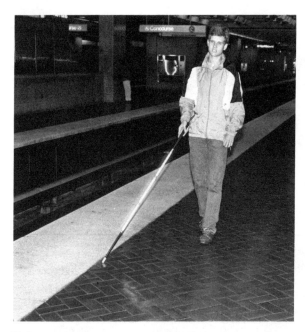

Using constant-contact technique while walking parallel to the platform edge is effective, but there is a danger of knocking other people over with the cane.

tracks and go slowly forward by keeping the cane in constant contact with the platform surface until the cane detects the edge or the different texture of the warning strip. Ask them to describe this texture, and then allow tactile exploration of the strip. They can extend their canes forward on the strip until the tip drops off; this procedure will give them an idea of the width of the strip. Students should practice locating the strip and the platform edge until they perform with confidence and self-assurance. Make certain that they do not position themselves on the strip.

Immediately after completing this training to identify the platform edge and the warning strip, begin instruction in platform identification and orientation. Have students locate the wall at the bottom of the last step of the stairway leading to the platform. Tell them to square off and start to find the platform edge or warning strip. After locating it, they should be able to return to the wall, then turn to the right or left, trail several feet, square off from the wall, and locate the edge and strip again. Students should follow this

After locating the platform edge, travelers should stand back away from the edge while waiting for the train.

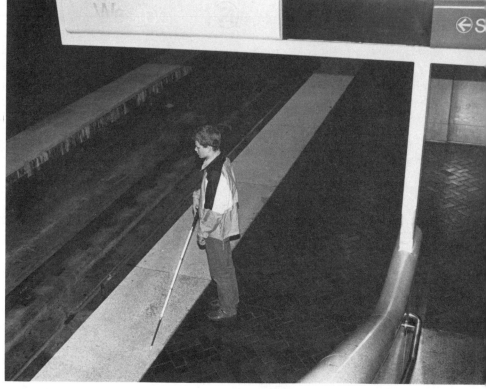

Walking Safely on Platforms

The following guidelines can be used by orientation and mobility (O&M) specialists in training blind and visually impaired students to walk safely on platforms:

SINGLE-TRACK PLATFORMS
Objective: To teach the proper procedure for walking on a single-track platform.

PROCEDURE
Method 1
1. The student stands on the platform.
2. The student locates the wall.
3. The student uses the cane to trail the wall and to walk from one end of the platform to the other.
4. While walking along the platform, the student locates the following: maps, benches, phones, elevators, steps, and escalators.
5. The student repeats steps 1-4 until he or she feels comfortable.
6. The student describes the platform.

Method 2
1. After the student gets off the stairs, escalator, or elevator, he or she turns and locates the warning strip near the tracks.
2. The student keeps the cane in contact with the platform to follow the warning strip across the length of the platform.

DOUBLE-TRACK PLATFORMS:
Objective: To teach the proper procedure for walking on a double-track platform.

PROCEDURE
1. The student stands on a double-track platform parallel to the warning strip.

2. The student moves the cane several times and identifies the seam between the regular textured surface and the warning strip.
3. The student proceeds, walking more slowly and keeping the cane in constant contact with the platform surface, following the warning strip. The student's feet should not be in contact with the warning strip at any time.
4. The student walks the entire length of the double-track platform and back several times, keeping the cane in constant contact with the platform surface.
5. If someone is in the student's pathway, the student asks to be excused and passes in front of the individual while staying off the warning strip, or walks around the individual and away from the tracks and then locates the warning strip and continues walking.
6. When a train pulls into the station, the student stops walking when he or she hears the train approach and steps away from the warning strip. Depending on the student's individual preference, he or she may maintain the present line of travel or turn to face the train. After the train has departed from the station, the student locates the warning strip and continues walking.

Note: These methods are used with platforms that have warning strips like the ones in Atlanta. They should be used only by individuals who possess excellent balance, gait, and texture discrimination skills with a cane.

procedure until they are sure they are oriented to the platform. (See "Walking Safely on Platforms.") They should use the procedure to determine when they are on a double-track platform. However, on a double-track platform, students will not locate a wall when they turn and walk away from the tracks. Instead, they will cross the island and locate another warning strip and platform edge. When students

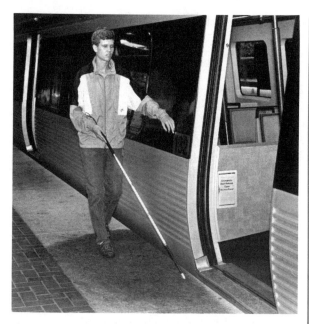

To orient oneself to the outside of a railcar, one should combine hand trailing with the use of a cane to trail the train.

become proficient in identifying double-track platforms, they should be able to walk safely in these areas.

Continue platform lessons with a session on auditory training for determining one's position in relationship to the train in a system. The length of the trains generally remains constant. Place students at the end of the platform where the back of the train stops, and have them listen to get a sense of the length of the train. Next, position them near the center of the platform so they can listen again as trains pass. When a train stops, they should be able to identify their position in relation to the front, middle, or back of the train. Repeat this procedure several times from various locations on the platform until they demonstrate good auditory localizing skills.

Another method for determining one's position is to relate the positions of the stairs, elevator, and escalator to the position of the train. Students should be familiar with the location of public conveyances and the station's architectural features. For instance, they know they can use the stairs to get to the plat-

form. Have them identify their positions in relation to the train. Repeat this procedure, using the escalator and elevator. This method can be used in several stations to determine if there is a way to correlate the locations of the stairs, elevator, and escalator with that of the train. If a correlation does exist, students can then preplan where to sit on the train. This strategy in turn helps in planning a route for exiting from the next station or for transferring to the next train. When waiting on a platform, students can stand with their backs against a wall, sit on a bench, or stand next to the warning strip.

Boarding the Train and Selecting a Seat

The following guidelines can be used by orientation and mobility (O&M) specialists in training blind and visually impaired students to board and select a seat on the train:

Objective: To teach the proper procedure for boarding and selecting a seat on the train.

PROCEDURE
1. The student listens for the door to open or for sounds coming from inside the train.
2. The student walks and locates the railcar with a cane, turns, and walks along the railcar, trailing the car with the cane.
3. The student's free hand trails the railcar and locates the rubber strip on the door edge.
4. The student detects an opening on the railcar with the cane.
5. The student extends the cane into the railcar and pushes the cane tip down to locate the floor.
6. The student slides the cane toward the feet to locate the space between the platform and the car.
7. The student steps into the railcar.
8. The student selects a seat near a door on the side of the train from which he or she wishes to exit.

Identifying Single-Track and Double-Track Platforms from Inside a Railcar

The following guidelines can be used by orientation and mobility (O&M) specialists to teach blind and visually impaired students to identify single-track and double-track platforms from inside a railcar:

Objective: To identify single-track and double-track platforms from inside a railcar.

PROCEDURE

1. The student and instructor sit on a train.
2. When the train stops at a station, the student identifies the side of the train on which the doors are opening by using cardinal directions. In Atlanta, when the train is traveling west and the door opens on the north side, it will open to a single-track platform; when the door opens on the south side, it will open to a double-track platform.
3. The student exits the train and establishes whether he or she is on a single- or a double-track platform.
4. The student reenters the train, proceeds to another station, and repeats steps 1-3.
5. The student repeats steps 1-4 until he or she performs with confidence and self-assurance.

On the Train

The next steps in the training program involve procedures from becoming oriented to the train itself and cover boarding and exiting, seat selection, and intercom use. These lessons need to be performed either in a train yard or at a station where the train is not in motion for a period of time. When orienting students to the outside of a railcar, instruct them to use the cane to trail the train in combination with hand trailing (i.e., using the fingers to follow the car's surface). At each opening, the cane should be inserted and lowered to clear the area to determine if the opening is a doorway or the separation between cars. This procedure should be repeated until the entire train has been explored.

The exiting procedure mirrors the boarding process. For effective orientation to the inside of the train, the perimeter of the area should be explored. (See "Boarding the Train and Selecting a Seat.") Inside the train, students can practice getting information directly from the conductor by using the intercoms inside the train.

It is important that students practice everything learned up to this point. They should be able to take the train independently from one station to the next, starting near the station entrance and finishing after they have become familiar with the second station. This lesson will indicate the areas in which further training is needed.

Toward the end of the lessons in rapid rail training, students should be instructed to associate certain door-opening patterns with single-track or double-track platforms. Guidelines on how students can learn to do this from inside the railcar will be helpful here. (See "Identifying Single-Track and Double-Track Platforms from Inside a Railcar.")

Following these step-by-step strategies for orientation to Atlanta's rapid rail system has routinized the training program and led blind and visually impaired persons to self-assured and safe travel. These lesson plans and whatever variations the O&M specialist must make in them offer a starting point and a proven approach to mass transit instruction.

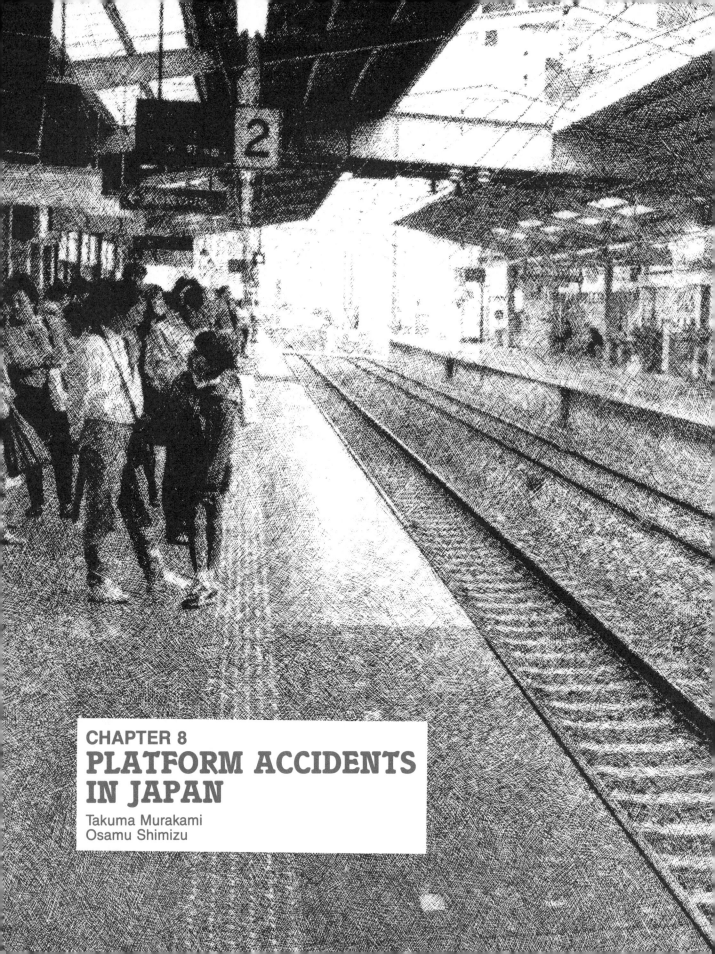

CHAPTER 8
PLATFORM ACCIDENTS IN JAPAN

Takuma Murakami
Osamu Shimizu

About 40 percent of Japan's population is concentrated in urban areas such as Tokyo and Osaka. Tokyo alone, with more than 11 million people, has approximately 28,000 legally blind persons using mass transit to commute to work, go to school, or pursue personal business or pleasure. People who are visually impaired or who are totally blind constitute another sizable group that depends on trains. Some of these blind and visually impaired travelers have had orientation and mobility (O&M) training, but the majority have not. As in other metropolitan areas, accidents have been reported among blind and visually impaired passengers.

A Study of Platform Accidents

The Tokyo subway system has two major types of train platforms: single-track platforms with a track on one side and double-track platforms with tracks on each side of the platform. Most platforms in Tokyo are double-track platforms. For example, of 29 stations on the Yamanote Line, which makes a loop through Tokyo, 27 (93%) are double-track platforms. These platforms are generally elevated 3½ feet from the railroad tracks. As in other mass transit systems, the double-track platforms pose the greatest danger for blind and visually impaired travelers.

As long ago as 1965, tactile warning tiles in the form of braille blocks were developed to make travel safer for blind and visually impaired passengers. (See "How Japan Accommodates Its Bus Travelers"

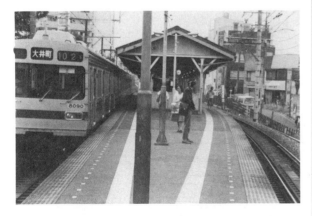

A majority of the platforms in Tokyo's subway system are double-track platforms.

in Chapter 6.) They were installed on sidewalks beginning in 1967 and on train platforms in 1970. The tactile warning tiles can be found throughout Japan, not only at bus stops and train stations, but on roadways and crossings, in public offices, and in agencies for blind people. In the Yamanote Line, for example, 26 platforms have tiles that are approximately 1-foot square and 3 platforms have 6-inch-square tiles. Tactile warning strips run the length of the platform about 3 feet from the edge. Tiles can also be found at the head or foot of many staircases and escalators. However, the pattern, shape, material, and method of installation of the tiles are not standardized. In spite of a number of studies undertaken to determine the best type of tactile tile, O&M specialists and their blind and visually impaired clients still must deal with unsolved problems in the use of these blocks, particularly how to apply cane technique to them (Murakami, Aoki, Taniai, & Muranaka, 1982). Although the introduction of tactile tiles, along with other systemwide improvements, has considerably expanded the potential for safer and more efficient travel for blind and visually impaired riders in Japan, serious accidents have occurred.

In 1983, a study was conducted to help understand the actual conditions surrounding life-threatening falls from train platforms by blind and visually impaired travelers. It was designed to examine the number of accidents involving falls from train platforms, analyze the causes of individual accidents, and present information that would help prevent them.

The study was conducted entirely through direct interviews with 54 visually impaired persons who had experienced falls from train platforms. All the participants in the study were residents of the Tokyo and Osaka metropolitan areas, were between the ages of 18 and 62, and had visual acuities ranging from total blindness to 20/100. Some of the main questions in the interview focused on the personal characteristics of the subjects, the number of years they had traveled independently, whether or not they had received mobility instruction, the number of falls they had experienced, and the types of platforms from which they fell.

Results of the Study

Among the 54 subjects, 23 fell once, 15 fell twice, 8 fell three times, 5 fell four times, and 3 fell five times. None fell more than five times. The total number of falls experienced by all subjects was 112.

The subjectively judged direction of movement on the platform at the time of each fall was included in the study. Blind and visually impaired travelers move parallel to the edge of the platform, perpendicular to the edge of the platform (facing the tracks), or in other unspecified directions. Among the 112 accidents suffered by the 54 subjects, 78 (70%) involved movement parallel to the track and platform edge. Twenty-two accidents occurred while subjects were walking toward trains to board them, moving perpendicularly to the edge of the platforms. Twelve of the accidents involved other lines of movement that were unclear.

Causes of Accidents

Some conclusions may be drawn from the accidents reported in the study. Specifically, in spite of the installation of tactile warning tiles, there seem to be few reliable clues to help blind and visually impaired travelers when they are walking along the length of the platform. Auditory clues usually related to the direction of the sound of other travelers' footsteps, as well as the sounds of station announcements and arriving and departing trains. But these clues are easily affected by environmental conditions. Even after establishing their direction of movement, blind and visually impaired travelers have a strong tendency to veer when trying to walk in a straight line across an open space with no obstacles.

There are, moreover, many obstacles on the platform, such as pillars, benches, newsstands, and moving passengers. In a recent experiment, a rectangular obstacle was placed either squarely or angularly in the path of subjects in order to measure their deviation from the expected line of travel after having negotiated their way around the obstacle. The results indicated that reestablishing an original line of direction after negotiating a way around an obstacle is almost impossible for a blind or visually impaired traveler who is using only directional cues from the obstacle itself (Tanaka & Shimizu, 1985). Maintaining a line parallel to the edge of the platform while traveling the length of the platform requires concentration. Therefore, a traveler walking a straight line or negotiating obstacles may be unable to detect the drop-off when he or she nears it.

The degree of danger accompanying a fall from the platform can also be considered in relation to the arrival and departure times of trains. Broken bones and bruises are the main injuries from falls that occur when no train is at the platform (except immediately before a train arrives). The danger of being hit by a train is minimal.

Falls that occur when a train stops only for a short time or just before a train begins to move are ex-

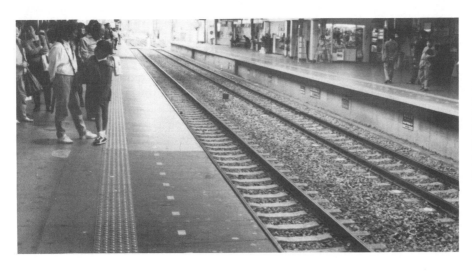

Many orientation and mobility specialists believe that improved cane techniques can increase the rate of drop-off detection and prevent platform accidents.

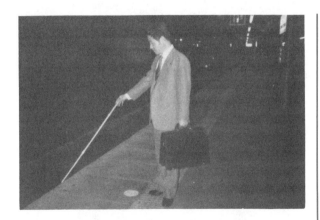

For some travelers, falls from the 3-foot drop-off in the Tokyo subway system can be caused by inadequate platform-edge detection techniques.

tremely dangerous. When a train is at the platform, the spaces between the cars always pose a danger to blind and visually impaired riders, who may mistake a space for an open door. In the study, a rather large number—5 of the 22 accidents that occurred when the subjects were walking toward the train—were falls in the spaces between the cars.

Falls sometimes occur immediately before an express train passes through the station or when a stopped train departs. In these cases, rescue is extremely difficult, and the chance of being struck by a train is very high. In some stations, there are open areas alongside the track or escape areas under the platform. Falls can take place in a location, however, where there is no safe place to escape from an oncoming train.

Only 20 percent of the 112 falls surveyed occurred while a traveler was waiting at the platform edge. In general, if travelers facing the platform edge pay careful attention, they can detect the drop-off. If it is assumed that the edge of the platform can be detected by using good cane techniques, it seems obvious that the number of falls in this category reflects the use of inadequate technique. However, this conclusion is questionable, particularly in view of the study results showing that falls happen even to those with a lot of travel experience. Yet professionals believe that improved cane techniques can increase the rate of drop-off detection and therefore

decrease the number of accidents occurring when blind and visually impaired riders are trying to board a train at the platform.

Many more elements are involved in accidents in addition to poor cane techniques. In the study, some other causes emerged, including mistaking the platform at which a train arrived or the time when a train might arrive at one of several platforms, confusing the sound of passengers' footsteps and incoming trains from other platforms with the sounds on one's own platform, engaging in overreliance on a sighted or a dog guide, and being bumped or pushed by other passengers on the platform.

Possible Solutions

An understanding of the basic causes of accidents and of the problems underlying those accidents can help transit authorities and O&M specialists analyze possible solutions. Some measures have been suggested as a result of this study: an extension or improvement of the textured tiles' installation, safety gates between cars, and the construction of closed platforms, which is considered an ideal solution. The expansion of O&M training for rapid rail travel would also undoubtedly reduce the accident rate. Blind and visually impaired individuals not only need to develop improved cane techniques but also to receive training in and to practice the other strategies that O&M specialists can offer.

At the same time, O&M specialists can act as mediators in effecting further changes and modifications in transit systems to ensure safer travel for their clients. Everyone concerned must recognize that, unlike a stumble at a street curb, even one misstep on a train platform can be deadly.

References

Murakami, T., Aoki, S., Taniai, S., & Muranaka, Y. (1982). Braille block on roads to assist the blind in orientation and mobility. *Bulletin of the Tokyo Metropolitan Rehabilitation Center for the Physically and Mentally Handicapped*, 11-24.

Tanaka, I., & Shimizu, O. (1985). Accuracy of reestablishment of the direction after negotiating an obstacle in blind mobility. *Nat. Rehab. Res. Bull. Jap.*, No. 6.

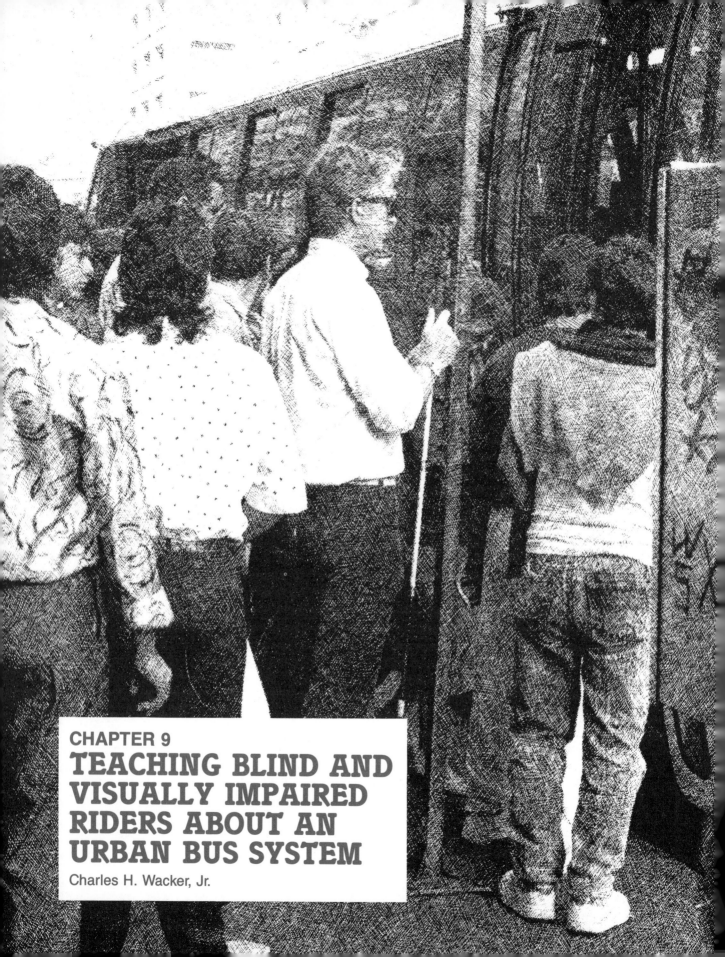

CHAPTER 9
TEACHING BLIND AND VISUALLY IMPAIRED RIDERS ABOUT AN URBAN BUS SYSTEM

Charles H. Wacker, Jr.

The Los Angeles bus system is a good example of a vast and complex urban bus system. The typical Los Angeles bus rider spends an average of 1 1/2 hours daily on the bus and may need as many as three transfers. As many as 1.8 million people ride over 2,280 miles via 241 bus routes every day (RTD News Bureau, 1986). They are served by the Southern California Rapid Transit District bus system

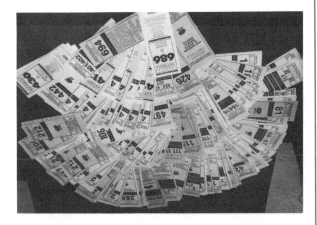

As reflected in the variety of tickets and transfers shown here, the Los Angeles bus system is a vast and complex network with as many as 241 routes.

(RTD)—the fastest-growing public transit system in the United States. Its ridership increased by 41 percent in 1986, so that it now carries 23 percent of the total Los Angeles population.

Large-City Problems

For blind and visually impaired travelers, size and scope of a system present a basic challenge but in no way reflect the full range of difficulties that must be overcome. In a county that is divided into 12 principal trading areas over 4,080 square miles in which there is no central business, shopping, or recreation area, traveling by mass transit can be complicated. Few buses take the traveler directly from point of origin to destination, necessitating transfers to buses either within the system or to the 100 other routes served by connecting bus lines. Transfer point locations can be crowded and noisy, and different buses often arrive simultaneously. With numerous bus stops on their routes, bus drivers do not give

verbal cues routinely, making it difficult for blind and visually impaired travelers to gauge where they are in relation to where they want to go.

Except for express buses, which use the freeways, buses travel on congested city streets. One must usually board near the beginning of the route to obtain a seat. Only orthopedically impaired passengers are specifically accommodated. To further complicate travelers' attempts at orientation, six different types of buses are used interchangeably, including double-deck and articulated (i.e., bend-in-the-middle) buses. On some of these, one enters at the front door and exits at the middle door. Others have only one door for entering and exiting. Seating arrangements also vary, and on the double-decker,

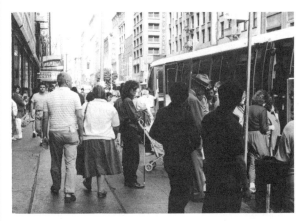

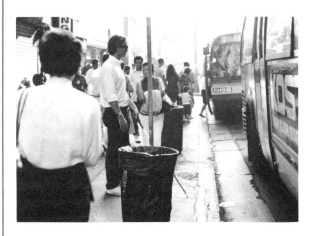

Bus stops that are crowded and noisy or used by different buses simultaneously are a source of confusion for blind and visually impaired bus travelers in large cities.

there is an upstairs seating layout with which to become familiar, plus, of course, the stairway to negotiate.

To meet changing situations, the bus authority must often add or delete routes, change bus numbers, or reroute buses. These changes naturally cause difficulty for blind and visually impaired travelers, in terms of both traveling and gathering information. Although there is a bus information hotline for disabled persons, it is heavily used and there are often long delays in reaching an operator.

Of the 2,500 buses in daily operation, many are older models that break down, resulting in delayed passenger transfers to other buses or the elimination of scheduled runs. Disruptions such as these pose problems for a rider with a set plan for making connections. In addition, weekend service is sometimes curtailed, making it necessary for a traveler to memorize a separate set of schedules and to make adjustments in travel time.

These are some of the specific problems encountered by blind and visually impaired travelers in Los Angeles. Although much has been done to facilitate bus travel, many improvements have little impact on travelers who lack the necessary functional vision to see and utilize them. Those with low vision suffer further difficulties when they, too, must rely on the sighted public for assistance.

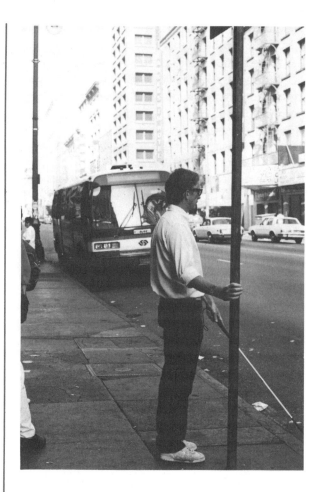

A lack of clear landmarks to signal the location of bus stops can cause blind and visually impaired persons to wait at the wrong stop.

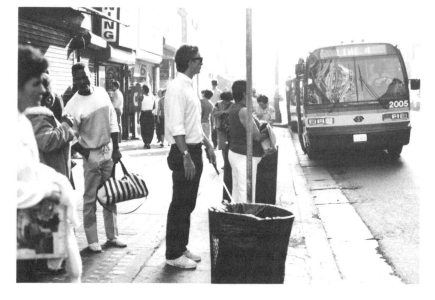

Workable Solutions

Many solutions to the difficulties of public transportation in Los Angeles have worked for blind and visually impaired travelers over the years. Although there are no infallible, universal answers that can be applied to all situations and all individuals, most of the solutions have broader applications beyond the Los Angeles area. If they can work in a vast and congested system, they can have satisfactory results almost anywhere.

It is important to recognize that in trying to improve bus travel for blind and visually impaired travelers, the orientation and mobility (O&M) curriculum must address and include three groups: blind and visually impaired bus travelers, bus company personnel, and the sighted public. An initial mobility evaluation is key to a practical prognosis of a blind or visually impaired individual's success as a bus traveler. Appendix 4 provides one sample of many available mobility evaluation checklists. An evaluation consists of a useful vision assessment that determines how much and how effective a person's functional vision is for travel and reading under various lighting conditions. Once the person's functional vision has been established, his or her conceptual and directional understanding of independent movement—that is, north and south, up and down, perpendicular and parallel, diagonal and opposite—needs to be examined. A trip around the block, starting at one point and returning to the same place, unescorted and following certain verbal cues given in advance by the evaluator, can verify this skill level. Finally, an evaluation of an independent bus trip, including route planning and bus information gathering, can substantiate skill level and signal basic problems to be dealt with in subsequent training.

An individualized bus training program deals with specific emotional, psychological, and performance difficulties encountered or imagined by a blind or visually impaired traveler. It must combine the mapping of a person's travel plans for the future and the evaluator's prognosis for independent bus travel for that person. It may involve extensive repetitive training in certain aspects of bus travel, such as gathering information, making transfers, and obtaining cardinal directions at specific corners. Such a program also means helping the person learn to interact with the sighted public and transit staff to solicit assistance and information. Depending on the person's needs, it may have to address how to maneuver around various structures with a dog guide. The development of the individualized lesson plan depends on an initial and extended evaluation but is also affected by unanticipated problems evidenced in the field training program. Some general rules for bus travel are outlined elsewhere in this chapter (see "Basic Tips for Training Blind and Visually Impaired Students for Bus Travel") and in *Orientation and Mobility Techniques: A Guide for the Practitioner* (Hill & Ponder, 1976).

Group Seminars

The generalized phase of bus travel training deals with the challenges mass transit presents for all blind and visually impaired travelers. These problems can be examined through group seminars on mobility conducted by an O&M specialist, representatives of the transit authority, and a rehabilitation agency staff psychologist, and through workshop field trips taken by the trainees as a group to one or more of the transit district's centers and to a bus information center. Ideas exchanged during seminars and field trips can be reinforced in the daily lesson plan for each trainee.

The seminars provide a place where excellent information exchanges on bus travel can take place and where trainees can find sounding boards for their trainees' feelings. The seminar facilitator should be an O&M specialist who may introduce a topic for discussion or encourage trainees to share their ideas and talk about their various experiences. Over the years, every conceivable personal problem encountered by blind and visually impaired travelers has been shared. Travelers have discussed getting their canes stuck in the door of a crowded bus and having the bus drive off, leaving them stranded on a corner without their canes. They have described their anxiety in asking sighted assistance, their trauma when taken past their stops, their fear of being robbed, and the hostility of other passengers.

Basic Tips for Training Blind and Visually Impaired Students for Bus Travel

PLANNING THE BUS ROUTE
Before starting out on a bus trip, a blind or visually impaired student should be able to plan his or her travel route by soliciting information about schedules and routes from the bus company. The following information should be solicited:
1. Time schedules, including specific information on bus schedule changes, such as those taking place during holidays and on weekends;
2. The number or name of the bus;
3. The exact location of bus stops nearest the student's point of travel origin, destination, and transfer points; and
4. Information regarding the use of transfers.

LOCATING BUS STOPS
The student should be familiar with the general characteristics of bus stops:
1. Bus stops may be located at the corners of intersecting streets and busy streets, or in the middle of a block, before or after the bus crosses perpendicular streets. In some areas, bus stops may be located only every few streets.
2. Bus stops usually have benches, shelters, or poles.

LOCATING THE FRONT DOOR OF A BUS
To locate the front door of a bus, the student should be able to do the following:
1. Localize sound clues, such as engine sounds and opening doors, that indicate the position of a bus.
2. Find the curb with a cane, and then check the distance to the side of the bus to gauge its distance from the curb.
3. Locate the door by trailing the bus either by hand and/or by using a cane.
4. Determine whether the door is at the front or the rear. It should be kept in mind that on city buses, the front door is usually located between the front wheel and the front bumper. On school buses the door is usually located behind the front wheel. School buses usually do not have rear doors.

BOARDING THE BUS
The following procedure should be followed when boarding a bus:

1. Ask the driver the number or name of the bus.
2. Hold the cane with the left hand so that the right hand can be free to hold the handrail and find the farebox.
3. Deposit the fare and request change. If a transfer or a pass is used, hand either one to the driver.

FINDING A SEAT
The following steps can be described to a blind or visually impaired traveler for finding a seat on a bus:
1. Tell the driver where you want to get off and ask him or her to let you know when you are there. Ask for a transfer, if necessary, and ask if there is an empty seat behind the driver or next to the door.
2. Proceed with the cane in your left hand and use the right hand to trail the overhead handlebar as you proceed to the vacant seat.
3. Check laterally along the front edge of the seat with the cane shaft to determine if there is room to sit down.
4. Keep track of where you are on a bus route by listening for clues and landmarks.
5. Check with the driver occasionally to find out if you are nearing your destination. This will also remind him that you are there.

EXITING FROM THE BUS
The following steps can be described to a blind or visually impaired traveler exiting from a bus:
1. Proceed to the front rail of the bus before the bus stops if you are on the driver's side or in the back of the bus.
2. Use the left hand on the front rail to maintain balance while getting off the bus. If you are seated next to a door, you should hold the pole at the edge of the stairs and stand and face the stairs before the bus stops.
3. With the cane in the right hand, step down, check the path for obstructions and try to locate the curb. Check for obstructions again, step up, and proceed.

If seminars are properly conducted, the participants can share before a peer group the anxieties, fears, difficulties, and joys they face as mass transit travelers.

From a practical standpoint, the seminars enable a review of checks and balances in mass transit, such as ensuring proper exits and transfers. What action should be taken if one passes one's stop? How can a passenger keep a bus driver aware of his or her presence and destination without causing antagonism? Discussions can cover the relationship between time and distance in bus travel and how to conceptualize these intangibles in terms of realistic route planning and implementation. Route planning can be done conceptually through timed

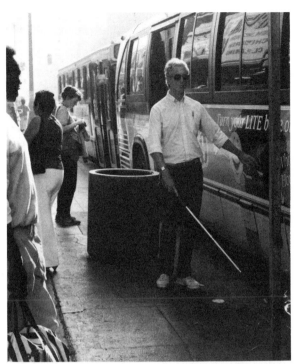

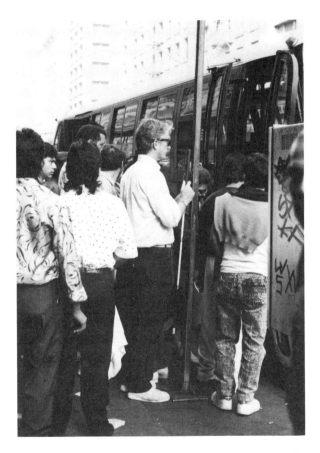

Learning how to deal with problems such as crowding, making transfers, and obtaining a seat are some of the topics discussed at group seminars for travelers.

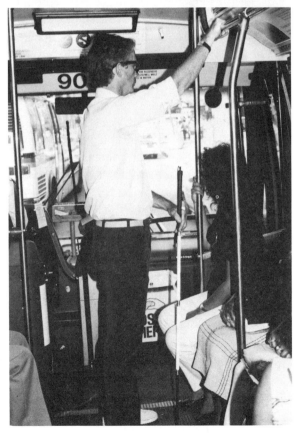

movements from one building to another and by comparing one person's route with another's.

Seminars should deal with the following problems: crowding; seating; making transfers; identifying oneself as a legally blind individual, including dealing with the visibility of one's cane or dog guide; soliciting recorded information about buses on the transit company's special telephone line; and understanding emergency procedures and precautions for safety and security. For example, knowing that most buses have a closed-circuit surveillance television system helps lessen a hopeless, panicky feeling when confronting a potentially frightening situation.

Representatives of the transit company's customer service department should be invited to attend the seminars periodically to answer questions and discuss changes, improvements, additions, problems, and solutions. They can provide immediate feedback for trainees on any aspect of bus travel that is of personal or group concern. Through them, workshop field trips to bus garages can be organized in order to orient trainees to the configurations of different models and styles of buses and their various features, such as their seating arrangements; exits and entrances; and special equipment, such as wheelchair lifts and variable platforms at the door that lower to the curb level. Transit representatives can also arrange for the group to visit a bus information center so that trainees can see the methodology and equipment used to handle incoming calls.

A psychologist can conduct several seminars throughout the year to handle problems relating to stress, anxiety, and the feelings of isolation of blind and visually impaired travelers trying to function in the rushed sighted world of bus travel. There is plenty of material for discussion here, including the problems of physical contact with strangers that is experienced when asking for assistance to cross streets; anger and frustration at not being heard when asking directions or eliciting other information from the sighted public; fear of being pulled instead of led through a crosswalk or around an obstacle; and the need to terminate unwanted attention and pity. The O&M specialist can contribute to the seminar by conducting role-playing sessions and engaging clients in desensitization experiences. Sighted assistance is integral to successful independent bus travel in many cities, and blind and visually impaired travelers should be able to communicate appropriately with the public. They must be able to accept help without reservation or resentment and know how to use it effectively. This point should be emphasized in seminars and reinforced in the field. An excellent resource on group mobility seminars is Blakeslee's (1980) discussion in the *Journal of Visual Impairment & Blindness*.

Bus Personnel and the Public

Successful bus travel for blind and visually impaired riders depends heavily on what bus company personnel and the sighted public know and think about the blind person they see on the bus or waiting at the curb. How will they treat this individual in a confrontation or in a casual encounter? The solutions to many problems lie in improved communication skills.

Seminars, tours, and meetings are needed with bus drivers and the public on a regular basis to explain blindness and visual impairment. For example, bus drivers as a group may adopt a patronizing attitude toward blind or visually impaired bus riders to disguise any uneasiness they may feel. Some drivers may stop the buses illegally and physically escort blind travelers on and off the buses as though dealing with mute invalids. Others may pretend not to see visually impaired travelers and may drive away, as happened in the case of a traveler who had the bus door slammed in his face after his cane got stuck in the door.

These reactions occur because some drivers believe they, not the company, are personally liable for the safety and security of their passengers. They become nervous and tense; normal job stress is compounded if they are afraid they will forget something, like calling out stops.

Bus security officers may have the same feelings, because they may perceive a blind person as someone who may become the helpless, immediate prey of a lurking criminal. In the view of some sighted people, there is something exceptionally vulnerable about a blind or visually impaired man or woman alone on a downtown street, in a crowded bus, or in a noisy depot. This fallacious attitude either drives the sighted individual to compulsive acts of over-protection or to the opposite extreme of fear of con-tamination and liability by association.

In regard to such issues, it is the responsibility of O&M specialists, along with their clients, to educate the public and bus company personnel. They need to interact with and include these groups in their orientation and training programs. Information brochures from the bus company's home office may help, but it is the instructor and the client who have to break the barriers of misinformation and prejudice through what they say and do on the street, at the bus stop, on the bus, at the transfer point, and in the depot.

Bus service in urban areas probably will remain congested, complex, and difficult in the foreseeable future. But bus travel for blind and visually impaired travelers anywhere can offer independence, free-dom, and the chance to participate fully in the community.

References

RTD News Bureau. (1986). Facts at a glance. *Los Angeles County Yearbook.* Los Angeles: Board of Supervisors.

Blakeslee, R. (1980). Group mobility seminar. *Journal of Visual Impairment & Blindness,* **74**(9), 357-359.

Hill, E., & Ponder, P. (1976). *Orientation and mobility tech-niques: A guide for the practitioner.* New York: American Foundation for the Blind.

MOBILITY EVALUATION CHECKLIST
APPENDIX 4

This checklist is to be used in determining the need of an incoming client for mobility training. The checklist is a comprehensive means of measuring a client's achievement level at the time of evaluation in preparation for training for travel in mass transit.

Because incoming clients may have received various levels of training prior to evaluation and have various degrees of functional vision, the orientation and mobility (O&M) specialist may choose to evaluate only those areas that are relevant to the individual client. Final evaluation regarding the client's competencies will be determined by all O&M specialists evaluating the client and will be submitted in a single report.

CLIENT _____ DATE _____

FUNCTIONAL VISION _____ YES _____ NO

DESCRIBE _____

_____

_____

I. Indoor, Campus, and Residential Travel

YES NO

YES	NO		
____	____	1.	Walks with a sighted guide in various situations.
____	____	2.	Locates objectives by trailing the wall with the back of the hand.
____	____	3.	Locates objectives visually.
____	____	4.	Uses visual clues indoors.
____	____	5.	Travels indoor routes utilizing visual information.
____	____	6.	Locates objectives and protects self by using the lower hand and forearm technique.
____	____	7.	Protects self by using the upper hand and forearm technique.
____	____	8.	Determines line of travel by squaring off from a straight surface.
____	____	9.	Determines line of travel by using a parallel surface.
____	____	10.	Seats self in various types of chairs, placing the cane in a safe, accessible position.
____	____	11.	Retrieves dropped objects.
____	____	12.	Uses visual clues outdoors.
____	____	13.	Travels outdoor routes utilizing visual information.
____	____	14.	Uses optical aids to read addresses.
____	____	15.	Uses optical aids to read street names.

		16.	Sees obstacles in the path.
____	____	17.	Sees drop-offs ahead.
____	____	18.	Protects self by using the diagonal cane technique.
____	____	19.	Uses the touch technique indoors.
____	____	20.	Uses the touch technique outdoors.
____	____	21.	Locates destinations by trailing walls with a cane.
____	____	22.	Locates and operates door mechanisms.
____	____	23.	Ascends stairs with a cane.
____	____	24.	Protects self by locating stair drop-offs with a cane.
____	____	25.	Descends stairs with a cane.
____	____	26.	Uses sound to aid orientation.
____	____	27.	Uses touch to aid orientation.
____	____	28.	Enters a car.
____	____	29.	Locates destinations by shorelining.
____	____	30.	Uses the touch-and-drag technique.
____	____	31.	Corrects a veer after crossing an open area.
____	____	32.	Uses compass directions for orientation.
____	____	33.	Travels to all buildings on campus from any location.
____	____	34.	Plans the safest, most direct route to any building on campus.
		35.	Understands the following basic concepts:
____	____		A. Streets
____	____		B. Sidewalks
____	____		C. Corners
____	____		D. Intersections
____	____		E. Stop signs
____	____		F. Stop light control
____	____	36.	Distinguishes the sidewalk from a street that has no curbs.
____	____	37.	Determines traffic location, distance, and direction of movement by listening when crossing streets.
____	____	38.	Crosses simple intersections.

II. Business Travel

		1.	Uses visual information while traveling in a complex business environment
____	____	2.	Distinguishes traffic light colors.
____	____	3.	Reads "walk/don't walk" signs.
____	____	4.	Uses optical aids to read bus destination signs.
____	____	5.	Uses near vision optical aids to read personal transit maps.
____	____	6.	Uses optical aids to read wall maps.
____	____	7.	Uses optical aids to read rapid rail signage.
		8.	Crosses complex intersections:
____	____		A. Oblique intersections
____	____		B. T-intersections

(continued on next page)

YES	NO		
____	____	9.	Solicits and controls aid with poise.
____	____	10.	Negotiates irregular sidewalks.
____	____	11.	Negotiates streets without sidewalks, but with curbs.
____	____	12.	Negotiates streets without sidewalks or curbs.
____	____	13.	Locates specific destination on blocks.
____	____	14.	Travels in areas that have obstructions, such as parking meters and lampposts.
		15.	Functions within a business establishment:
____	____		A. Adjusts cane technique
____	____		B. Solicits aid when necessary
____	____		C. Comprehends the layout of store environments
____	____		D. Makes purchases
____	____	16.	Uses escalators.
____	____	17.	Uses elevators.

COMMENTS _____

_____

_____

_____

SOURCE: Adapted from a mobility checklist from the Foundation for the Junior Blind, Los Angeles, California.

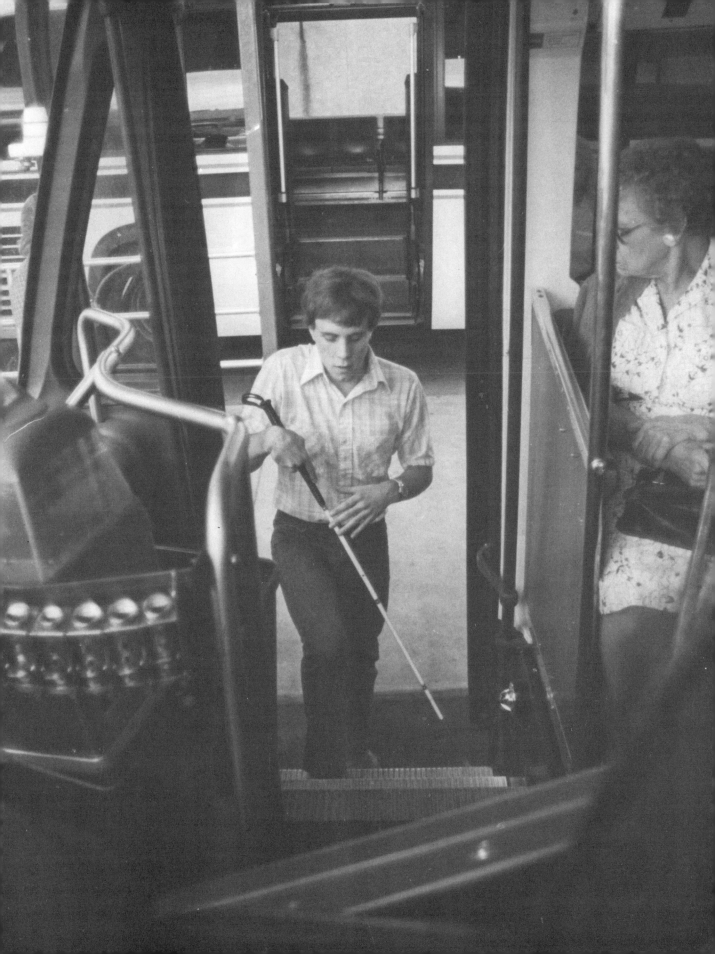

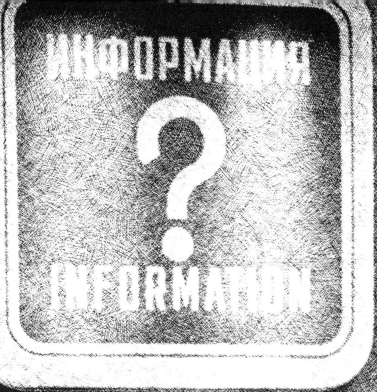

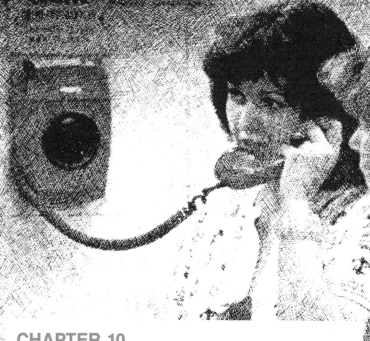

CHAPTER 10
A THREE-PRONGED PLAN FOR SOLICITING TRAVEL INFORMATION

Steven J. LaGrow
Robert O. LaDuke

Since the development of systematic orientation and mobility (O&M) instruction in the 1950s, the training process for improving a visually impaired person's ability to travel has had to keep pace with a fast-moving and fast-changing society. Books such as Naisbitt's *Megatrends* (1984) have pointed out major changes that have had an enormous impact on society. The ongoing process of decentralization is a good example. Starting in the early 1950s, the mass movement of people from central core communities to the suburbs resulted in three important developments that have had a profound effect on blind and visually impaired travelers.

First, the suburban environment was developed primarily to be aesthetically pleasing and largely accessible by automobile. The lack of grid patterns and walkways for pedestrians seriously hampered access to the wide range of commercial facilities that followed people to the suburbs. Second, public transportation was not readily available, nor even seen as a need, for many of the newly built communities. (Fortunately, short-haul lines and private carriers have alleviated this problem to some extent.)

The third major element in decentralization was the dispersion of businesses along major traffic arteries. Business growth did not occur in a clearly defined business area but in plazas and malls stretched along busy streets. The factors that favored this growth, such as availability of parking spaces, the accessibility from major streets, and space for large, multiple-product retail facilities, created special problems for pedestrian customers, which certainly included the blind and visually impaired population. O&M instruction has had to help blind and visually impaired travelers deal with momentous developments such as these.

Additional Effects of Societal Change

The national penchant for intercity and interstate relocation has had an additional impact on blind and visually impaired persons. Census Bureau figures indicate that almost 40 million people changed their places of residence between 1983 and 1984 (U.S. Bureau of the Census, 1986). The average American moves once every 6½ years, or about 11 times in a lifetime. There is no reason to believe that blind and visually impaired persons do not change their residences as often as their sighted peers do. Thus, the nature of the instructions given them for adapting to their environments must accommodate ever-changing travel needs.

Still another influence on mobility instruction has been a national trend away from family and institutional help to a greater reliance on the individual's own abilities. Probably one of the earliest examples of this change was the lobbying by blind and visually impaired students and their parents for local education in the early 1950s. As a result of this activity, these children were among the first to be mainstreamed. Society now expects persons with special needs to meet those needs within their home communities, but it neither expects nor encourages them to work. Institutionalized disincentives to employment have left many competent persons with disabilities without work. To fill their time meaningfully and pleasurably, blind and visually impaired persons—and others with disabilities—must be provided with extensive access to their communities.

There is a growing recognition that disabled people have a right to such access. Evidence for this can include the deinstitutionalization movement, increased physical accessibility in public facilities, the presence of auditory devices in theaters, the existence of closed-caption television and talking computers, and various other subtle yet significant improvements.

Finally, there has been a vital change in the potential for travel by blind and visually impaired persons as a result of the increased availability of professional O&M instruction. From the advent of systematic travel training provided by the Veterans Administration in the 1950s to the development of the first university programs for mobility instructors in the following decade, to the current state of the art, there has been an expansion of the expectations for travel among virtually all segments of the blind and visually impaired population. To meet their needs, instruction has been broadened to provide them with more information than was ever necessary in the past.

Need for Instruction and Information

Moving efficiently in and around both familiar and unfamiliar environments requires a systematic procedure for obtaining precise location and travel information. This includes learning the exact location of a destination, relevant transit information, and information or directions relating to walking to the destination, if walking is necessary.

The exact location of a destination can best be obtained by calling the destination to ask for instructions on how to get there and finding out if bus or other public transportation is required. Transit information can then be solicited from the transit system to get as close to the destination as possible. If more information is needed to walk from the bus drop-off point to the destination, it may be obtained from designated public offices. In most cities, public officials can give precise information relating to traffic-light location, the availability of sidewalks, and the nature of the intersections to be crossed.

A procedure for soliciting information has been designed to enable blind and visually impaired people to gather complete objective travel information from the primary sources just described. Components of this process have been used by many blind and visually impaired travelers, but a systematic approach was first developed by Robert Savage at the Michigan Rehabilitation Center for the Blind in Kalamazoo, Michigan. It has been modified and used in many cities around the country. It has also been used with sighted mentally retarded students and visually impaired college students, as well as with a full spectrum of clients seen in rehabilitation centers for blind persons. Currently, it is being used with graduate students in O&M at Western Michigan University.

If a traveler is to plan the best route to a given destination, he or she must have complete and precise information. That is the primary goal of learning the procedure outlined in the following discussion.

Finding the Destination

It is important to first find out where a place is located, particularly in relation to the nearest corner, and whether bus or other public transportation is necessary. One begins by calling the destination to get this information, which must include the address, the name of the closest intersecting street, and directional corner information.

The Address

An address does not always indicate the exact location of a place. It does, however, provide a means of verifying the quality of the information obtained. The address should enable a traveler to determine the name of the street on which the destination is located, the side of the street on which the destination is located, and the relative distance of the destination to a specific corner. If any discrepancies are found, one must request clarification to determine if there are inaccuracies in the information provided. If the person providing information is found to be in-

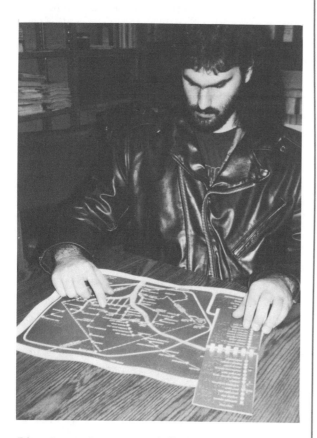

Planning one's route carefully before going on a trip can ensure success.

accurate when giving compass directions, for example, a traveler can change his or her information solicitation strategy by asking if the destination is located on the right or left side relative to some place with which both the traveler and the person are familiar.

Most places are located on the streets corresponding to their addresses. However, sometimes a store can have entrances on more than one street, or a business located on a corner can have its main entrance facing the primary commercial street and its official address on the intersecting street. It is important to ask which street the main entrance faces, even when the address is known.

Corner or midblock location can also be anticipated on the basis of street address. It is not uncommon, however, to find that streets do not always continue through the entire city. Therefore, numbers may split midblock rather than at the corner. This split occurs where the intersecting street would be if it existed in this particular location. It is also important to know if the odd-even sequence changes sides when a dividing street is crossed.

Directional Corners
The corner nearest to the traveler's destination must be identified among the four corners in a standard intersections to provide the traveler with a means of planning the most efficient route. Descriptions of a corner's location in terms of direction (i.e., north/south and east/west) are specific and exact. They are not relative, like descriptions using the corners of right and left. As a result, directions may be used to specify a destination's exact location and to plan a route to it, regardless of the location from where the person is traveling.

Landmarks and Clues
A traveler can further specify the location of his or her destination by determining those features that distinguish it from all other buildings or locations. For example, it could be the second building south of a particular intersection, and its entrance could be the first door south of an alley. Greater specificity can be obtained if something distinct is known

---

Key Questions for Soliciting Location Information

The following questions will help blind and visually impaired travelers solicit specific information about the location of their destinations:

1. What is your address?
2. What street does the entrance face?
3. On which side of the street are you located?
4. Are you near a corner? If not, which corner is nearest to you? The corner of [name of street that the destination's entrance is on] and what other street?
5. What direction are you from [name of the intersecting street]?
6. How far [name the direction] are you from the corner [number of doors, buildings, sidewalks, stores]?
7. Is there anything distinctive about your building or entrance that would help me know that I have arrived?

---

about the entrance or storefront. For persons with functional vision, information about color or contrast can prove extremely helpful.

In general, a simple series of questions can be used to elicit the exact location of a destination when one is calling the destination for information. (See "Key Questions for Soliciting Location Information.") The traveler needs to figure out how to get to the corner nearest to the destination from his or her starting point. If this is not immediately apparent, he or she may wish to call a source of public transit information.

Using Mass Transit
In addition to needing information about their given destination, blind and visually impaired persons need to obtain information about relevant mass transit in order to plan a route for an outing. The strategy presented here specifically relates to city buses, but

it can be adapted to meet the peculiarities of other forms of public and private transportation.

Basic Information

In order to obtain basic information, travelers need to call the transit office and inform the operator from where they will be starting and where they wish to go. In doing this, they should tell the operator the intersection closest to the starting point and closest to their ultimate objective. Directional corner information is not needed at this time, for it will probably only cause confusion. However, information concerning the direction in which the bus will be traveling and the street on which it will be running is important. The traveler can then determine on which directional corner he or she will need to be in order

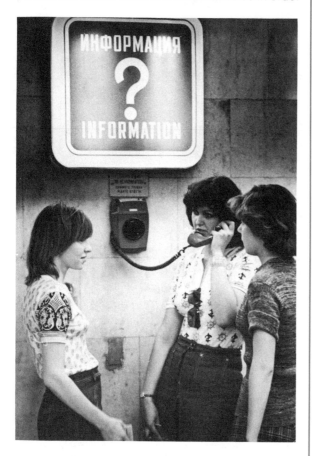

Information about mass transit can be obtained from telephone information services found in some transit systems, such as this one in the Moscow system.

to board the bus and on which corner he or she will be when leaving the bus. Directional corner information is crucial when planning the route for walking.

Directional Corners

Directional corners can usually be determined if one knows the direction in which a bus is traveling. Two basic principles are helpful here. First, buses are always loaded and unloaded on the right side of a street. Therefore, one can determine the side of the street on which to board the bus. For example, if the bus is traveling north, it will stop on the east side of the street. Second, if a bus stops before an intersecting street to avoid blocking an intersection, one can determine the side of the intersecting street where one can expect to catch the bus. For example, if the bus is traveling north, it will stop on the south side of the perpendicular street. Knowing these two facts, the traveler can expect the bus to stop at the southeast corner of the intersection. Buses do not always stop before an intersection, however, and one should always check with the transit telephone operator and the driver to be sure.

Transfer Points

When they make inquiries concerning bus travel, blind and visually impaired people may sometimes find that they need to transfer to another bus route. When this is the case, they need to gather a variety of information. They should determine the direction in which the bus will be traveling when it arrives at the transfer point, the street on which the next bus will be, the direction in which the second bus will be traveling when it leaves the transfer point, and the direction in which the bus will be traveling when it arrives at the required destination. They also need to determine which bus to catch originally, where to catch it, where to disembark to transfer, which bus to transfer to, where to catch it, and where to disembark to walk to their desired destination. In addition, they also need to know where to catch their return bus, whether transferring buses will be required, and where to transfer if necessary. Finally, routes may vary by time of day. Travelers should let the transit

Key Questions for Soliciting Bus Information

The following questions will help blind and visually impaired travelers solicit specific bus information to get to their destinations:

1. I am at the corner of [provide the intersection from which travel will begin] and wish to go to the corner of [provide the intersection nearest the destination] at [particular time of day]. Can you tell me which bus I can take?
2. On what street will the bus be traveling when I catch it?
3. In which direction will the bus be traveling?
4. Will it stop before or after the intersection?
5. Will I need to transfer buses? If yes:
   a. Where must I get off to transfer?
   b. On what street will the bus be when I get off?
   c. In which direction will the bus be traveling when I get off?
   d. Where do I catch the bus to which I transfer?
   e. On what street will it be?
   f. In which direction will that bus be traveling when I catch it?
6. Where can I get off so that I will be as close to [name the intersection nearest the destination] corner as possible?
7. On what street will the bus be when I get off?
8. In which direction will the bus be traveling when I get off?
9. Where will I be in relation to my destination [name the intersection nearest the destination]?
10. Where can I catch the return bus (and where is that in relation to where I get off)?
11. Which bus is it?
12. On what street will it be traveling when I catch it?
13. In which direction will the bus be traveling when I catch it?
14. Will the bus stop before or after the intersection?
15. Will I need to transfer buses?
16. Where is the bus stop nearest the corner of [name the intersection to which you are returning or where you wish to get off]?
17. On what street will I be when I get off?
18. In which direction will the bus be traveling when I get off?

telephone operator know when the trip will be taken and make sure the information provided will still be valid if plans are changed.

Usually, a series of specific questions can elicit complete information from the transit office. (See "Key Questions for Soliciting Bus Information.") By following the procedures outlined in this discussion, it is possible for a blind or visually impaired person to assemble enough information to expedite travel by bus from a specific departure point to the bus stop nearest his or her destination.

Walking There

Gathering information related to walking requires a little more work on the part of the traveler. The questions to be asked cannot be predicted as easily as can those presented earlier, and the sources of reliable information vary. Information on walking may be needed if a bus does not drop the traveler within a few blocks of his or her destination or if the destination is located in an unfamiliar environment. Often, sufficient information can be obtained from the transit telephone operator and verified by a call back to the destination. If this strategy does not work, or if the information provided is not clear, the blind or visually impaired person may wish to contact some other source of information.

In some cities, departments such as those dealing with public works and traffic engineering can be relied on, but police and fire departments as well as other agencies may have information available. Through such sources, blind and visually impaired travelers can find out where the destination sought is in relation to the bus stop, whether there are sidewalks along all the streets to be traveled, and if there is any street or road repair under way. Travelers can usually find out how many blocks they must travel in any given direction to reach their destination. In addition, the department of traffic engineering can be called to determine where traffic or pedestrian lights are located along any particular route, what the relative volume of traffic is like on the streets, whether the streets run one way or two ways, and, if they are one way, the direction in which traffic flows.

Persons answering the phones in departments called for information require some in-service training. Without training, people tend to provide far too much information. (See "Adaptations for an Accessible Transit System" in Chapter 5 and "Advocating in Behalf of Visually Impaired Travelers" in Chapter 6.) Experience has shown that most persons in public offices are quite willing to help. In fact, many persons take pride in their ability to provide accurate information rapidly. People calling for information should exercise discretion, however, because excessive inquiries can irritate those providing the service.

Additional information can be obtained from pedestrians and operators of businesses in the area. When using these sources, it is always necessary

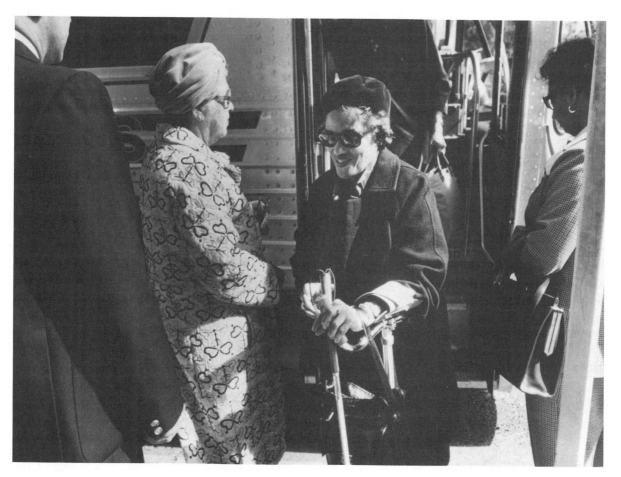

While on route, visually impaired travelers may find it helpful to verify with other passengers information they have obtained beforehand.

to verify the information given by referring to known streets and landmarks. If one is traveling in a known environment, it is easier to ask for directions from pedestrians in front of major stores and at intersections.

Information should be obtained in such a manner that it can be organized in segments. The logical segments of routes usually correspond to the junctures where changes of direction are required. Segments are usually best organized when they include the number of blocks and the direction to be traveled, the name of the street that will be traveled on, and the directional corner, landmark, or objective marking the completion of each segment or route. In this fashion, the traveler can organize a fairly complex route into a number of discrete segments.

All the information gathered will enable the blind or visually impaired person to gain access to a constantly changing environment. The development and use of more structured approaches to information gathering have been necessitated by rapid societal changes over the past 30 years. The methods described here ensure that complete information can be obtained to help blind and visually impaired people travel independently in both familiar and unfamiliar environments.

References

Naisbitt, J. (1984). *Megatrends: Ten new directions transforming our lives* (6th ed.). New York: Warner Books.

U.S. Bureau of the Census. (1986). *Geographical mobility, March 1983-March 1984.* (Population Reports Series P20 No. 407.) Suitland, MD: Author.

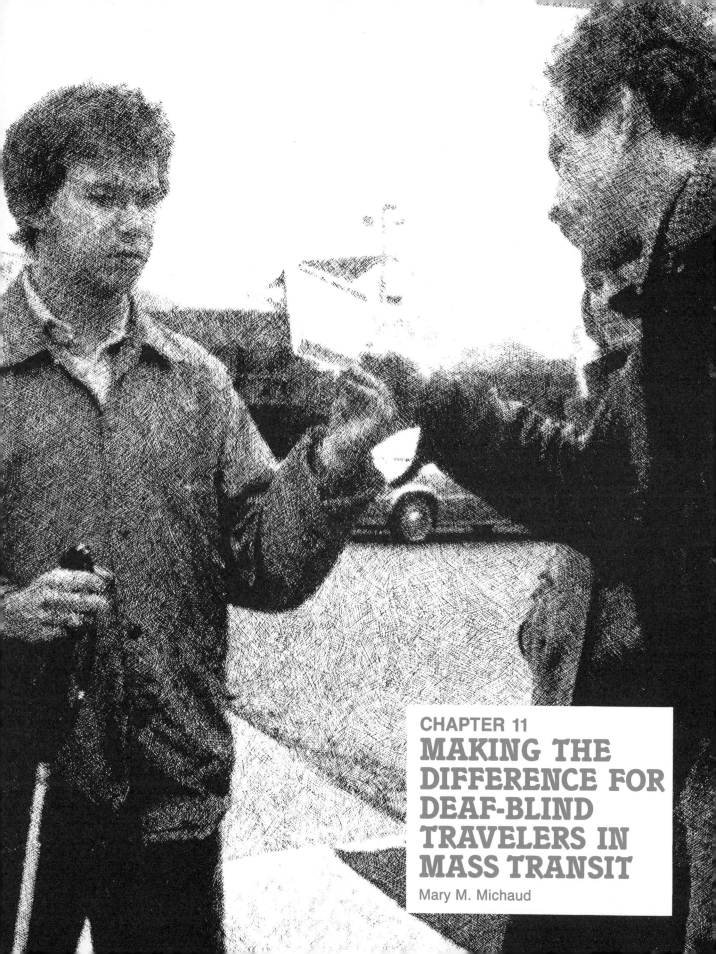

CHAPTER 11

MAKING THE DIFFERENCE FOR DEAF-BLIND TRAVELERS IN MASS TRANSIT

Mary M. Michaud

Many deaf-blind individuals travel to and from work by bus, train, or subway every day. They face the same difficulties and challenges that have been described for blind and visually impaired travelers using public transportation. Perhaps they face even more.

Issues in Mass Transit

Specific areas must be addressed and given priority attention by orientation and mobility (O&M) specialists to help deaf-blind people overcome problems and achieve success in mass transit travel. Two of these focus points are communication and alternative sensory input.

Communication

How will a deaf-blind person who needs information communicate with the public? Skills in this area that need to be evaluated and developed include the client's expressive and receptive means of communication as well as his or her ability to use these means effectively to obtain assistance, direction, or information. The crucial—and often deciding—factor in a deaf-blind person's choice of method of communication in many travel situations is which method is most understood and accepted by the public. A deaf-blind traveler may be quite skilled in Tadoma, a method of tactile lipreading, for example, but if the other person objects to having a stranger's hand on his or her face, the deaf-blind person may have to reconsider the usefulness of this method and choose another strategy. (See "Choosing Receptive and Expressive Methods of Communication: Guidelines for the Orientation and Mobility Instructor.")

Alternative Sensory Input

Because they are without the ability to hear and localize sound, deaf-blind travelers need to develop other sensory systems to assist them in identifying clues and landmarks, taking directions, and orienting themselves to their environment. Textures, vibrations, wind, temperature change, and other such factors all begin to play a primary role. A deaf-blind person must be able to identify and effective-

Choosing Receptive and Expressive Methods of Communication: Guidelines for the Orientation and Mobility Instructor

When choosing any of the receptive or expressive communication methods, certain factors should be considered. Is the method:

- *portable?* Can the device be easily stored in a pocket or handbag? Is it heavy or bulky? Remember, deaf-blind persons must carry this with them at all times.
- *durable?* If prewritten cards are being used, are they laminated? Do electronic communication devices require careful maintenance? What about weather conditions—will rain or sleet adversely affect the device used?
- *practical?* How practical and convenient to use is this device for the situation?
- *speedy?* Can communication be established quickly and smoothly, or is the communication method generally slow and time consuming? (This is a consideration in situations in which tight schedules and transfers are a factor.)
- *limited in the length of the message that can be generated?* Will the message most likely be short (three or four words), or will it be longer? In-depth information is difficult to receive with methods such as a braille card. (The Tellatouch, however, allows for lengthier messages.)
- *known or accepted by the public?* Is the general public aware of this communication method? Will a brief orientation be done first? How likely is it that it will be accepted by the people with whom the traveler comes in contact?

ly use sensations prompted by these factors to gain vital information about the environment. Learning the techniques or strategies that have worked well for other deaf-blind clients using public transportation is a challenge for both the instructor and the student.

Level of Communication and Travel Skills, by Group

The four categories of deaf-blind persons have the following levels of communication and travel skills:

I. Congenitally Deaf-Adventitiously Blind (Persons with Usher's syndrome)
   A. Communication Skills[a]
      1. Has fair to excellent American Sign Language skills.
      2. Uses some home signs and gestures.
      3. Has limited English-language skills.
      4. Has no braille skills.
   B. Travel Skills
      1. Is an experienced traveler.
      2. Relies heavily on visual cues that may be increasingly ineffective.
      3. Has no previous experience with such elements as mobility training and low vision aids.
      4. Often does not understand his or her eye condition and its effect on mobility.
      5. Often does not want to have anything to do with the instructor or the mobility program.

II. Congenitally Blind-Adventitiously Deaf
   A. Communication Skills[a]
      1. Has excellent English-language skills.
      2. Has excellent speech.
      3. Has good to excellent braille skills.
      4. Is resistant to tactile communication—wants to rely on remaining hearing, which may be progressively ineffective.
      5. Talks to avoid awkwardness of receptive communication.
   B. Travel Skills
      1. May or may not be an experienced traveler.
      2. Has had mobility training in the past; is familiar with mobility devices; is often a cane or a dog guide user.
      3. Relies heavily on auditory cues that may be increasingly ineffective.
      4. Is unable to localize sound (traffic, doors opening, people speaking).

III. Adventitiously Deaf-Blind
   A. Communication Skills[a]
      1. Has excellent English-language skills.
      2. Has good to excellent speech.
      3. Has no braille skills.
      4. Is unable to use tactile means of receptive communication.
   B. Travel Skills
      1. Is an experienced traveler.
      2. Has good visual memory.
      3. Has no previous mobility training; is not a cane user.
      4. Often does not travel at all; is in need of total mobility program.

IV. Congenitally Deaf-Blind[b]
   A. Communication Skills[a]
      1. Has little or no formal communication skills (such as speech, sign language, reading, and writing ability).
      2. Communicates through gestures, pictures, and visual demonstration.
   B. Travel Skills
      1. Has little or no independent travel experience; is often accompanied by parents or staff.
      2. Is a visual traveler; learns best through demonstration, pictures, and repetition.
      3. Often has had previous mobility training; uses cane for identification.
      4. Has difficulty handling unexpected situations or changes along a route.
      5. Has difficulty transferring and generalizing skills to new areas or routes.

[a]Communication skills categories are all derived from Wynne (1982).
[b]Refers to the rubella population. Because this population encompasses such a wide range of functioning levels, this group is delineated as those individuals who have the ability to travel semi-independently within the community.

A Look at the Population

In January 1987, the Register of Deaf-Blind Children and Adults maintained by the Helen Keller National Center for Deaf-Blind Youths and Adults listed and identified 11,000 deaf-blind individuals in the United States. This number was estimated to be only one-quarter of the actual population. A more realistic estimate would bring the number to a growing 40,000-44,000. Who are the people represented by these statistics, and what are their needs and abilities?

Because the members of the deaf-blind population are so varied in terms of ability and levels of functioning, it can be helpful to divide them into the following four categories to examine their characteristics and needs: congenitally deaf-adventitiously blind, congenitally blind-adventitiously deaf, adventitiously deaf-blind, and congenitally deaf-blind. Although it must not be forgotten that each person has individual needs, goals, and experiences, many deaf-blind persons display common characteristics, which allow them to be grouped in this manner. The common elements within each group relate to the communication skills or modes most often used and typical travel abilities and experiences. Knowing these elements can help the instructor plan more effective programs and teaching strategies. (See "Level of Communication and Travel Skills, by Group.")

In an attempt to discover whether people in one group within the deaf-blind population are more likely to be mass transit users than others, an informal assessment of the clients who have been seen at the Helen Keller National Center since 1980 was conducted. Table 1 shows the results of the assessment.

The assessment clearly showed that the majority of the deaf-blind population surveyed used public transportation; half of these mass transit users were clients with Usher's syndrome. Clients who had had rubella made up the second largest group. Those children who were part of the rubella epidemic of 1963-64 are now moving in steadily increasing numbers from the educational system into this country's network of rehabilitation services. It is estimated that

Table 1. Clients at the Helen Keller National Center Who Use Mass Transit

Category[a]	Percentage
Non-users of mass transit	40
Severely multidisabled Congenitally deaf-blind	25
Community travelers who travel to a limited degree (a mix of Groups I, II, III, and IV)	15
Mass transit users	60
Usher's syndrome (Group I)	30
A mix of Groups II, III, and IV, with rubella clients constituting the largest portion	30

[a]Group I=congenitally deaf-adventitiously blind; Group II=congenitally blind-adventitiously deaf; Group III=adventitiously deaf-blind; Group IV=congenitally deaf-blind.

SOURCE: Informal survey done by the author at the Helen Keller National Center for Deaf-Blind Youths and Adults, 1980-1986.

approximately 800 rubella children will be making this transition within the next five years (Olson, 1986). Mobility specialists can therefore expect to see more of this type of client in their caseloads. (For a description of clients at an agency serving multidisabled and deaf-blind persons, see "Multidisabled Blind and Visually Impaired Travelers.")

Factors Contributing to Success in Travel

Not all deaf-blind individuals reach a level of independent travel that enables them to use mass transit. Many travel quite well within familiar indoor environments. Others enter or get around the community, but not necessarily by public transportation. On the basis of an informal survey and discussions with mobility specialists, 10 factors have been identified as having caused a certain measure of success in the 60 percent of the deaf-blind travelers from the Helen Keller National Center who use mass transit. These factors are the following: some degree of remaining sight or hearing; ability to use tactile, proprioceptive, or cutaneous methods of input; good orientation skills; prior experience with public transportation; assertiveness, aggression, and the ability to use the public to advantage; ability to understand

Multidisabled Blind and Visually Impaired Travelers

Mastering travel in mass transit may be challenging for many blind and visually impaired individuals, but it becomes even more complicated when the individual has other impairments. At the Elwyn Institute in Pennsylvania, which has provided custodial care for 130 years but now offers comprehensive educational, recreational, rehabilitative, vocational, and daily living skills programs, blind or visually impaired travelers are often also multidisabled. This implies a different set of needs, skills, and limitations.

Although multidisabled blind and visually impaired students at Elwyn Institute may not have an immediate need for mass transit, receiving instruction for mass transit travel will prepare them for the future. In the case of individuals with multiple impairments who are unlikely to use mass transit independently, instruction may be limited to exposure and traveling with a sighted guide.

Depending on the nature of the person's impairments and skill level, some individuals will be able to use mass transit extensively and others will not. Some visually impaired mentally retarded persons may realistically be expected to learn only a few specific travel routes that entail mass transit. In such cases, the individual might be taught small portions of a route until he or she can put it all together and travel from starting point to destination and back.

Blind or visually impaired persons who use a wheelchair may require extensive training to be able to get around independently. Although they may not be expected to travel beyond the confines of the institute, they may use mass transit when accompanied by a friend or family member and therefore should be exposed to mass transit travel.

Some multidisabled persons have poor stamina because of medical complications and need to rest periodically as they travel. Others may have memory or other cognitive problems that require travel instructions to be put in either large print or braille, on cassette tape, or on a simple tactile map.

When dealing with persons with severe multiple disabilities, orientation and mobility (O&M) specialists have to determine whether a student can be allowed to travel independently and, if so, how independently. Although O&M specialists are accustomed to this responsibility, it becomes a more imposing task when the individual is mentally retarded. The possibility of a blind or visually impaired mentally retarded person getting lost when traveling alone is greater than with other clients. Contingency plans for what steps to take when someone is lost should be part of the instruction.

For many multidisabled individuals, independence in the community may be experienced for the first time during O&M training, and their own fears as well as those of their families must be confronted. These fears may stem in part from poor self-esteem, fear of failure, past negative experiences, or fear of the unknown. Parents may be uncertain about a child's ability to use mass transit or to deal with people, among other concerns. Direct service staff may possess fearful misconceptions about the client or about blindness in general. Lessons in utilizing mass transit can confront these fears and misconceptions and provide a format for positive, educational, and normalizing experiences.

Because of the varied cross section of individuals who have different impairments, O&M specialists must master many skills. Depending on the student or the client, the specialist may use any of a number of devices, such as prewritten cards, picturesymbol cards, a language board, a touch talker, sign language, or behavioral learning technique support devices. Specialists have to be creative, and they need to consult many other skilled professionals, including deaf-education teachers, teachers of the visually impaired, speech and language therapists, psychologists, physicians, case workers, residential counselors, physical therapists, and occupational therapists, when working with a blind or visually impaired multidisabled individual.

—*Chester Lubecki*

the choices available; independence and motivation; ability to communicate through speech; in congenitally deaf persons, good English-language skills; and ability to communicate with the public by two or more methods.

Degree of Remaining Sight or Hearing
Given the amount of information a deaf-blind traveler must gather and process about the environment, as well as the amount of communication with the public that is often needed during travel, someone without any remaining sight and hearing would find it increasingly difficult to negotiate the more complex systems of public transportation. Of the 154 clients surveyed who were able to use public transportation, two-thirds had remaining functional vision, one-fourth had functional hearing, and the majority had varying degrees of both. Only 20 were totally deaf-blind. All 20 were able to travel by bus. Only 11 were able to utilize commuter trains and only 2 used subways independently.

Ability to Use Alternative Methods of Input
Despite the fact that the majority of deaf-blind persons surveyed using mass transit have some remaining functional vision or hearing, these sensory modes often prove inefficient as a primary means of information gathering in certain environments or situations. For example, subway stations are so noisy that several deaf-blind individuals have stated that they have turned off their hearing aids when standing and waiting on the platform. At night, a person with Usher's syndrome is often unable to see the familiar visual landmarks he or she may use along a bus route during the day. For these reasons, it is vital that deaf-blind persons learn to assimilate and incorporate often-subtle tactile, proprioceptive, and cutaneous cues into their travel routines.

Good Orientation Skills
Many complaints heard from deaf-blind persons about the public transportation system center around huge, disorganized, and confusing systems whose characteristics are often inconsistent or irregular. A deaf-blind person must have orientation and

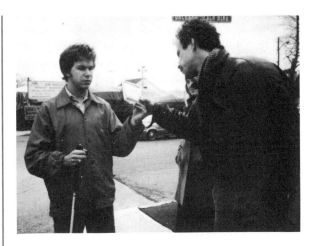

Deaf-blind travelers often have to seek assistance from the public by using prewritten questions.

problem-solving skills to deal with these complex, ever-changing environments.

Prior Experience
For the majority of deaf-blind people, prior experience with certain forms of public transportation plays an important role in the desire to use mass transit again. The confidence or level of anxiety experienced by a person, as well as any preference for a particular type of system, will be determined by that experience. For example, deaf-blind individuals who did not use the subway before losing their sight or hearing will often prefer using a bus. One client who used subways daily as she grew up preferred this means of transportation, for she was familiar with the individual stations as well as with the transit process, the pitfalls, and the risks.

Ability to Use the Public
It is clear that deaf-blind persons sometimes require assistance from the public, especially in travel environments where they have little control over the situation, such as when buses break down, schedules change, subways are delayed, or tracks are switched. Often, just identifying the correct bus at a terminal requires aid. In order to get information, directions, or help, a deaf-blind person must seek out willing (or unwilling) pedestrians, quickly estab-

lish rapport, make the person feel comfortable, and get the assistance required. To do this, he or she cannot be shy, soft-spoken, or naive. It takes an assertive, often aggressive personality to seek and obtain the vital information needed at that moment, especially when people are running to catch a bus or train or are unwilling or afraid to deal with strangers.

Although conductors and bus drivers can be helpful and willing to provide assistance, too often they are not available when needed. It is important, therefore, that deaf-blind persons know how to use the public to their own advantage. They must, for instance, know where people congregate. At one particular bus stop, people tended to stand in the doorway of a corner drugstore rather than at the bus stop itself. Although John, a deaf-blind person, stood by the bus stop sign, he knew where to go if he had a question or needed help. Similarly, in certain subway stations people gather at the bottom of the stairs leading to the platform. Knowing this kind of information will help a deaf-blind person know where to go should he or she need assistance.

Ability to Understand Available Choices

Like everyone else, deaf-blind travelers need to be able to make decisions, such as which route to take or whom to approach for help, on the basis of the options available. But in order to make decisions, they need to understand the basis for those decisions—that is, they need to understand the choices before them. For example, in one subway station that John used frequently, several newspaper stands were located on the platform. John assumed he could get information from the people behind the counter. Unfortunately, some of them did not speak or read English well. It is difficult enough to try to use an unconventional communication method with a stranger; it is particularly hard to determine if he or she speaks the same language.

The issue of identifying choices also relates to the need to approach appropriate pedestrians. In some cities, one is perhaps just as apt to meet some questionable characters as to encounter honest and helpful individuals. The presence of tattered or ill-smelling clothing or the smell of alcohol on a person may be a clue that it is best to seek another person's help. Also, a deaf-blind person must be aggressive enough to break contact when necessary. Unfortunately, one young deaf-blind woman was not able to make this distinction. She was able to travel independently by train to a train depot and communicate effectively, but she often approached for assistance mentally ill or homeless persons wandering in the station. Problems of risk and safety then entered the picture: These are other issues for deaf-blind people using mass transit.

Independence and Motivation

Mass transit can sometimes be the most difficult, complicated, and anxiety-producing forms of travel a person can encounter. Numerous variables are out of the traveler's control when he or she enters a transit system. In addition, the traveler must use a particular method of communication to elicit directions or information successfully. Yet, these major obstacles notwithstanding, 60 percent of the deaf-blind persons in the study were able to use mass transit. For many, a strong desire to be able to visit friends, get a job, or attend a social event or deaf club meeting was a factor in their success. For all, a desire for regained independence and self-respect was the key.

Ability to Communicate Through Speech

Thirty percent of the clients surveyed who used mass transit had understandable speech. Although this was not the case for the majority of the mass transit travelers in the survey, understandable speech appeared to have an effect on the level of travel the 30 percent were able to achieve. Approximately one-half were able to travel on the subway, which may be considered the most complex of mass transit systems. Of those clients without speech, only one-quarter achieved the same level.

Good English-Language Skills

It is important that deaf persons develop their skills in English as much as possible. American Sign Language (ASL), which is a deaf person's first language, is a language in and of itself and has its own grammatical structure, which is different from the grammatical structure of English. Because it is a visual language, not a written language, it may be difficult for deaf persons who primarily use ASL to write notes and follow written instructions.

Ability to Communicate by Two or More Methods

The number of communication methods deaf-blind persons are able to use successfully with the public will influence the level of independent travel they will achieve. Scott, a young deaf-blind man with excellent travel skills, is a case in point. Scott was trained with the Mowat Sensor and could complete complex routes, but his only means of expressively communicating with the public was with prewritten cards prepared by his instructor. When he lost or misplaced them, which was quite often, he was helpless. Consequently, Scott was never able to travel independently within the community, despite his excellent mobility skills. He always needed someone to accompany him for interpreting purposes.

The nature of the environment is a major consideration regarding the importance of communication skills. The more complex the environment, travel route, or travel system used, the greater the need for skills in various communication methods. Uncontrollable variables and unexpected changes often make it necessary for the deaf-blind traveler to supplement information, receive directions, or solicit assistance, all of which take a skilled communicator.

How can deaf-blind persons accomplish these tasks? How can O&M specialists help them develop the communication tools that will aid them in reaching their true potential? A closer look at possible methods of communication along with other factors influencing the instructor's choice of strategies will provide some answers for deaf-blind travelers.

Methods of Communicating with the Public

The broad topic of methods of communication can be divided into two subjects: receptive and expressive communication. Several means of receptive and expressive communication are used by deaf-blind individuals when they are traveling in the community and using public transportation. It is common for people to be skillful in one or some areas but not in others. Knowing which areas an individual needs strengthening in is crucial to effective programming.

Receptive Communication

Hearing. Receiving information from connected speech based on the ability to understand such speech, can be one of the most helpful methods of receptive communication. It does not require anything special on the part of the public other than, possibly, speaking louder or, in some cases, in lower tones. However, even those deaf-blind persons with the best hearing often find this method of input ineffective in some situations. Loud, extraneous noises, such as buses or subways pulling into a station, a radio or a street musician playing, or other people talking, can compete with the person speaking. All these elements can interfere with a deaf-blind person's ability to receive the messages he or she needs. The inability to localize sound can also make establishing contact difficult. A deaf-blind person may hear voices nearby but be unable to determine from which direction they are coming.

An important skill that deaf-blind persons must learn is the ability to express their needs at the beginning of a conversation, for example, by stating such messages as, "I'm hard of hearing. Can you speak louder?" "Could you please turn your radio down?" or "My right ear is better than my left." Information like this clarifies the situation for the public, prevents frustration that might arise from ineffective communication, and makes the "helper" more willing to assist.

Reading. Two-thirds of the deaf-blind clients in the Helen Keller National Center survey had some remaining functional vision, and reading signs, messages, notes, schedules, and notices was an all-important method of input for them. Low vision devices are often appropriate for people with functional vision. Carrying pen and paper is even more important for mass transit travelers. Many deaf-blind persons prefer to use a black felt-tip pen, often finding messages written in lead or ink difficult to read. In addition to a pen or marker, travelers also need something on which to write, and a small pocket notebook is handy and portable. Deaf-blind persons cannot expect someone else to provide supplies; they must take on that responsibility themselves.

It is vital that the instructor evaluate a person's language level and reading ability. A person with Usher's syndrome with limited English-language skills may have difficulty understanding a series of directions. If this is the case, instructing him or her to ask another person to draw a map may be a workable alternative. In addition, many rubella deaf-blind people are nonreaders. For them, focusing on pictures, survival words, or one- or two-word phrases may be effective. Many rubella clients, although unable to read, are able to match the name of a bus written on an index card with the sign on the bus.

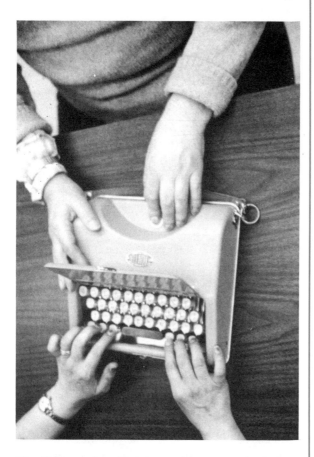

The Tellatouch, which is used by many deaf-blind travelers, has a typewriter keyboard that produces braille symbols.

Tellatouch. The Tellatouch is a small machine with a typewriter keyboard. As an alphabet key is depressed on the keyboard, the corresponding braille symbol is raised on the back of the device. To use the device, a deaf-blind person must know braille. Consequently, those most often familiar with this method of communication are congenitally blind persons. The Tellatouch is generally accepted by the public. Most people are familiar with typing, and the mechanical nature of the device appeals to many. Also, people in general are uncomfortable with the physical closeness and contact necessary with most other methods of receptive communication, and when the Tellatouch is used, physical distance can be maintained. It is not necessary for a pedestrian to touch a deaf-blind person directly when using the machine.

Tadoma. Tadoma is a method of tactile lipreading in which a deaf-blind person positions his or her fingers on the other person's lips, nose, jawbone, and neck. For some, it is a supplement to auditory input. Although some deaf-blind individuals are able to use Tadoma successfully, this method of communication is seldom taught or used today. Its biggest disadvantage is nonacceptance by the public. Few people are willing to have anyone, particularly a stranger, place his or her hands or fingers on their faces. One deaf-blind man in the survey who was quite skilled in Tadoma only used it with family and friends. He often chose to use other communication methods when traveling.

Print on Palm. In Print on Palm (POP), a person prints large block letters with his or her index finger on the palm of the deaf-blind person's hand. In general, the deaf-blind person must be familiar with print. This method can be used to determine quickly a train track number or the cost of a ticket or to receive short messages. Because it is a relatively slow means of input, it is not recommended for travel situations in which lengthier messages are needed.

Braille or Alphabet Cards. Braille or alphabet cards are pocket-sized, durable, laminated plastic cards with braille or raised alphabets. In using an alphabet card, the sighted person spells out his or her message by placing the deaf-blind person's finger on each letter individually. The braille card is easier to carry around but is slower to use than the Tellatouch. It is often used by clients just learning braille. The alphabet card is seldom used by most deaf-blind persons. Many prefer to use POP rather than to carry one more item around.

The Yes, Yes-No System. The yes, yes-no system is a communication strategy used by deaf-blind persons with intelligible speech. Leonard, a deaf-blind client, used this strategy frequently when traveling to and from work. He would tell a person that he was going to ask him or her a series of yes-no questions. If the answer was yes, he asked the person to tap his hand or shoulder twice; if the answer was no, to tap only once. No taps meant the person did not know. Using this strategy, Leonard was able to get important information regarding bus arrival times, schedules, changes, or delays.

Tactile Speech Indicator or Phone Listener. The tactile speech indicator (TSI) is an inexpensive telephone device called the phone listener that has been modified so that it can be used as a vibrotactile aid by deaf-blind people (Wynne, 1980). In it, a thin plastic disk is inserted over the telephone speaker's amplifier. The deaf-blind user places his or her fingers on the plastic disk to feel relevant signals, such as telephone rings, busy signals, or voices. The person using the device should possess usable speech so that he or she can ask questions over the telephone and receive appropriate answers, such as "yes," "no," or "I don't know," which come over the speaker as a single, double, or triple vibration (Cote, 1987). It is a handy device for calling a taxi or bus or a train station for schedule information.

Expressive Communication

When looking at various modes of expressive communication, some pertinent questions should be considered. Is this communication method one that can be independently and spontaneously generated by a deaf-blind person, or one that must be prepared by someone else? Can this method be generated during a trip, or must it be prepared beforehand?

Can the message be applied in several situations?

Whenever possible, the method used should be one that can be spontaneously generated by the individual, produced on the spot, and applied in several situations. This allows the client more flexibility when traveling independently. Methods that are limited in content or that must be prepared before a trip usually contain information specific to a particular route. These limitations could be a problem if a deaf-blind person finds himself or herself lost or faced with unexpected changes, delays, or rerouting.

Speech. Speech is a highly effective method of communication in most situations. One disadvantage, however, is that people often assume that because you can speak, you can hear as well. Bob, who had perfect speech, often chose to "turn off his voice" when riding the bus and to use prewritten cards instead, in order to avoid this misunderstanding. Many times, drivers had called out his stop on the assumption that Bob had heard them. Bob's prewritten card requested the driver to tap him when they came to his stop, alleviating this dilemma.

Buttons that read "I am deaf and blind" are often worn to clarify a situation. In Bob's case, when speech was used, Bob usually found it necessary to begin conversations with "I can't hear you. I'm deaf."

Writing. A variety of portable writing guides can be made by the instructor and used effectively by a client to write short notes or messages. Cutting three or four spaces out of the top of a checkbook cover and replacing the checks with paper cut to size makes a handy guide. Taking a plastic 8.5″ × 11″ writing guide and cutting it into three smaller guides makes the guide more portable. It should be remembered, however, that a client's skills and language level must be evaluated first to determine the most useful guide.

Prewritten Cards. Prewritten cards can take a variety of forms and are a widely used method of expressive communication. Rather than write a note again and again each day (such as a street crossing card), a deaf-blind person can type his or her message on an index card and laminate the card.

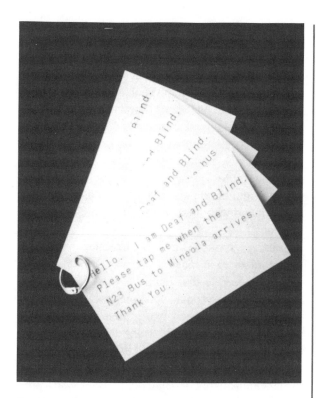

A prewritten series of cards cued to a particular bus route can help a deaf-blind person communicate specific information or requests to bus drivers and other passengers.

Prewritten cards, however, have their disadvantages. The messages are limited in content and therefore cannot be applied in several situations and cannot be added to or changed. Many cards are prepared for specific routes or specific situations. Nevertheless, those who are unable to write will depend solely on prewritten cards. When these cards are used, routes should be simpler; because public transportation is often limited to bus travel, fewer possibilities exist for errors, delays, or problems. Organization is an important factor in using prewritten cards. The following scenarios illustrate this principle:

- One man loosely placed his cards in his shirt pocket. When he reached for one, the others fell onto the train platform and into the trackbed.
- When boarding the 5:00 p.m. bus on a Friday afternoon, other passengers waited impatiently as Sue fumbled and searched her purse for the "right card."

- To cross the street to his bus stop, John took his street crossing card from his pants pocket. It was crumpled, torn, and barely readable. John apologized; it had gone through the wash with his pants that morning.

Clients will often have several cards for a particular route involving mass transit, or many cards for various routes. Organization is the key to the successful use of many different prewritten cards as a communication method. Cards can be organized into portable picture books, credit card holders, or small notebooks; placed on chains or card rings; or stored in an index file if the client is an extensive traveler. Color coding, brailling, and laminating cards can be useful organizational strategies. Clients should be helped to develop an organizational system that works for them. It can often mean the success or failure of their travel in mass transit.

The Loop Tape. A loop tape, or an answering machine tape that repeats its message, has been used to express simple messages or requests for help. (Tapes that can play messages 15, 20, or 30 seconds long can be purchased at electronic stores.) The tape recorder used in traveling should be small, portable, and water resistant, if possible. When the loop tape is set up and the tape recorder is turned on, the message will play over and over until the deaf-blind person gets the assistance he or she needs.

Picture Communication Books. Picture communication books can be used in many different formats, depending on the client's language level and visual ability. In general, a picture communication book is a method developed for any individual who requires an alternate, supplemental way to express or receive information. Picture-word or picture-phrase combinations can be created to communicate key points in a given situation. The size and complexity of the picture is an important consideration: pictures that are too busy or too small should be discarded. Pictures can be drawn or cut from books or magazines, or actual snapshots can be used. They can be in color or black and white. Every communication book is unique, reflecting each deaf-blind person's particular communication skills and needs.

Alternate Mobility Techniques and Strategies

How can deaf-blind people, without hearing as well as without sight, gather the information about their environments that they need to master mass transit? The number of strategies and skills available include the development and use of remaining sensory systems, the use of modified cane technique, and the use of electronic devices. A detailed examination of these and other techniques follows.

Use of Remaining Sensory Systems

A primary role in the way a deaf-blind person receives and gathers information is played by the proprioceptive, cutaneous (tactile and thermal), haptic, and, to a lesser degree, olfactory sensory systems. By placing greater emphasis on this area of training, the O&M specialist will be looking at the environmental clues and landmarks on which deaf-blind people often depend and certainly need in mass transit.

The Proprioceptive System. The proprioceptive system detects and compensates for such factors as surface changes (irregularities and conditions causing a shift in balance, such as the tactile warning tiles on platform edges), degree of elevation (gradients or drop-offs, such as a ramp leading into a station or the drop-off at the platform edge), and direction changes (curves or angles, such as a bus curving or turning at specific places along a route).

The Cutaneous System. Helen Keller described the importance of the cutaneous system eloquently:

> I think people do not usually realize what an extensive apparatus the sense of touch is. It is apt to be confined in our thoughts to the fingertips. In reality, the actual sense reigns throughout the body, and the skin of every part under the urge of necessity, becomes extraordinarily discriminating. It is approximately true that every particle of the skin is a feeler which touches and is touched (Harrity & Martin, 1962, p. 149).

Vibration, wind, temperature changes, and surface textures provide important bits of information for this system.

The cutaneous system has two main components. One is tactile and relates, for example, to the feel of wind or vibration as a train pulls into the stop or platform, as doors open and close quickly, or as people rush quickly along the train or subway platform. These cues can be used by a deaf-blind person to confirm a train's arrival. The other is thermal—and relates to natural and man-made temperature changes caused by sun, wind, and rain and heating and cooling systems, such as air conditioners or heating ducts. A deaf-blind person is able to feel the heat or cold as a train's doors open and close. This is a way to confirm that the vehicle is actually stopping to let people out, rather than stopping because there is a delay. To use this kind of information, many deaf-blind people will sit next to or stand near the door.

The Haptic System. The haptic system uses the body, hand, and cane to receive tactile information about the environment. This process can be the primary means of sensory input for deaf-blind persons. Therefore, the haptic system plays a major role in independent travel. Without auditory cues such as the sound of a bus or train pulling up, people's voices or footsteps moving in a certain direction, or a turnstile clicking to allow people in and out, a deaf-blind person may rely on trailing a wall or surface as an alternative. Doing so enables the traveler to maintain a line of direction; locate door entrances, intersecting halls, or walkways; and find important clues or landmarks, such as turnstiles, entrance gates, benches, or information and ticket counters. Difficulties may arise, however, if a deaf-blind person depends too extensively on trailing. Environments such as those found in subways, with large expanses of open areas and free space to cross with few tactile guidelines, may pose a problem through which the client and instructor need to work.

A deaf-blind person's sense of touch becomes finely developed as he or she relies on it more. It is the sense most often used to gather information as well as to communicate with others, and orientation to a new environment is a slow, often time-consuming process: hands are needed not only to explore the environment but to receive information and directions as well.

The Olfactory System. Use of the olfactory system consists of relying on both man-made and natural

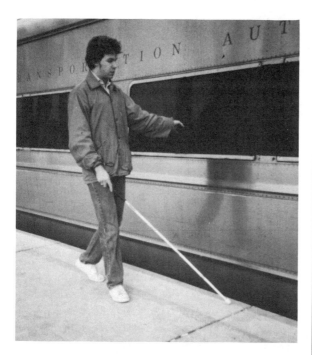

The constant-contact technique combined with hand trailing is particularly helpful to deaf-blind persons because they have to rely heavily on tactile input.

odors as cues. Man-made odors, like those emanating from a bakery or dry cleaning store on the same corner as the bus stop, and natural odors, such as those coming from a flower shop at the entrance to the subway station, provide important orientation cues. The olfactory system is often too unreliable to be used as a primary sensory input system, but it can be used to back up one of the other three systems just described.

Cane Techniques

Certain modified cane techniques are particularly helpful to deaf-blind persons. For many deaf-blind travelers, using constant contact techniques is a preferred method of cane travel. In the following comments, Fisk describes why it is a preferred method:

> During standard two-point touch technique travel, the cane tip. . . leaves the walking surface and breaks the tactual linkage. Allowing the tip to remain on the ground provides superior tactual feedback, resulting

in the detection of small surface discontinuities and precise location of walkway margins, with obstacle detection equal to that provided by the two-point touch technique and superior detection of vertical breaks in the walking surface. Drop-offs, sharp gradients, and blended curbs are detected earlier, thus improving reaction time, because the edge of the discontinuity may be contacted at any point of the cane arc, rather than just at its outer reaches (Fisk, 1986, p. 999).

These comments were based on a study using a blind-hearing population as the test group. The technique, however, proves doubly important for deaf-blind individuals who rely heavily on tactile feedback and information. The constant-contact technique is a method most individuals prefer.

In addition, many deaf-blind individuals also prefer to use special marshmallow-shaped cane tips. Fisk has explained the reason for this:

> The marshmallow tip's widely beveled circumference. . . facilitates its riding over irregularities and providing information about their presence and location without impeding progress. In combination, the constant-contact cane technique and the marshmallow cane tip allow the application of the long cane in such a way as to minimize sticking and maximize tactual feedback from the travel path . . . (Fisk, 1986, p. 999).

Electronic Devices

An electronic device highly appropriate for deaf-blind individuals is the Mowat Sensor, a hand-held ultrasonic obstacle sensor with a vibratory output.

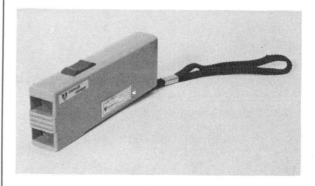

Because of its portability and capacity to detect obstacles, the hand-held Mowat Sensor is useful for many deaf-blind travelers.

Nevertheless, only 8 of the 154 mass transit users who were part of the study used this device. Varying reasons were given by deaf-blind clients for not utilizing the device more often, such as the need for maintenance and the need to recharge the unit. Some also had a sense that the extra information obtained was superfluous because they were familiar with the route they were using and the landmarks. Others felt they already had enough to carry, such as a cane, communication cards, writing guides, and tactile maps. Still others objected to the constant vibration from the device, which was caused by the presence of many people on the platform or at the bus stop. In the study, the sensor was not appropriate for mentally retarded deaf-blind persons who were not able to understand or interpret its signals or for those with remaining functional vision.

Despite some of the perceived disadvantages and limitations, the Mowat Sensor did have specific advantages and uses for the deaf-blind travelers using mass transit. It helped them maintain a line of direction by allowing them to shoreline without direct and constant contact with the wall, to follow people in line, to solicit aid, to locate people at the bus stop, to find open doors on a train or subway, to judge the space between the train and an open door, and to identify the arrival of a bus. These are just a few of its applications. Although the number of deaf-blind clients in the survey that chose and were able to use the Mowat Sensor was limited, the sensor's advantages as a mobility device are reason enough to make its use an important option in O&M training.

Additional Considerations

Certain information and techniques emerged again and again among the responses of the deaf-blind mass transit users surveyed. Three areas were mentioned regularly: the use of familiar versus unfamiliar routes, "following the crowd," and risk factors.

Unfamiliar Routes

Unfamiliar routes pose major problems for many deaf-blind persons. Self-familiarization to a new route, bus stop, or train or subway station is often a difficult and time-consuming process. Because there are few consistent landmarks or layouts in train or subway stations, it is almost impossible to transfer information about one station to another. In addition, the amount of sensory input available about new environments is limited for deaf-blind persons. Although they could ask people for information, ease of communication is an issue. Getting detailed feedback may be too time-consuming and too difficult to achieve when people who are rushing off to jobs or home are approached.

A majority of deaf-blind individuals, and even the most advanced travelers among them, will stick to familiar routes when using mass transit. As one person said, "In unfamiliar places, I ask for a guide. I get a lot of assistance. I'll ask for help at the time, but then later will follow up with a more formal, in-depth orientation to the route. To plan my communication strategies, such as the cards I might need, I need to be familiar with the route." For those who undertake self-familiarization, the ability to identify appropriate persons and develop systematic questioning techniques is a vital skill.

Use of Crowds

Following the crowd in mass transit situations is not often recommended by mobility specialists for students learning to travel independently. Pedestrians will not always make judgments that deaf-blind and visually impaired persons can rely on as safe, such as when it is appropriate to cross the street. Deaf-blind and visually impaired travelers are taught to think independently, and in most cases this is valuable. In certain situations, however, following the crowd has proved effective and accurate enough to use on a regular basis. In a busy subway or train station where there are one or two exits or entrances, deaf-blind persons often state that they are able to locate open doors or stairways into or out of the station by following the flow or direction of people. It is one situation in which relying on the volume of people is more helpful than harmful. One deaf-blind man exclaimed, "I couldn't swim upstream if I tried. Before I know it, I'm out the door, up the stairs, and into the street."

Risk Factors

Risk factors must receive special consideration when deaf-blind persons are traveling in certain environments, such as dark or isolated subway stations or infrequently used bus stops. It is more difficult for deaf-blind travelers than for travelers who can see or hear to determine or sense if they are in a potentially dangerous situation or if they are placing trust in an unreliable person. Safety is a vital issue. What can deaf-blind persons do to protect themselves? Here are a few suggestions that O&M specialists can pass on to their students:

- Travel in familiar areas only. Know where you are going and walk quickly and confidently.
- Take the bus rather than the subway.
- Take a longer route if necessary to avoid a dangerous neighborhood or stop.

- Do not travel alone. Travel with a known friend or colleague through a particular area.
- Do not wear an identification button conspicuously. Buttons with such messages as "I am deaf and blind" or "I am deaf and visually impaired" are often worn by deaf-blind persons as a means of getting assistance or clarifying their needs or disability (as in the message "I'm not ignoring you. I'm deaf"). As a rule, buttons are extremely effective—at street crossings or in supermarkets, for example—and they are frequently purchased by deaf-blind persons who wear them willingly. For some travel situations, however, such as nighttime subway travel or walks through high-crime neighborhoods, the instructor should recommend that the person not wear an identifying button openly. Buttons can be kept in a pocket and presented if

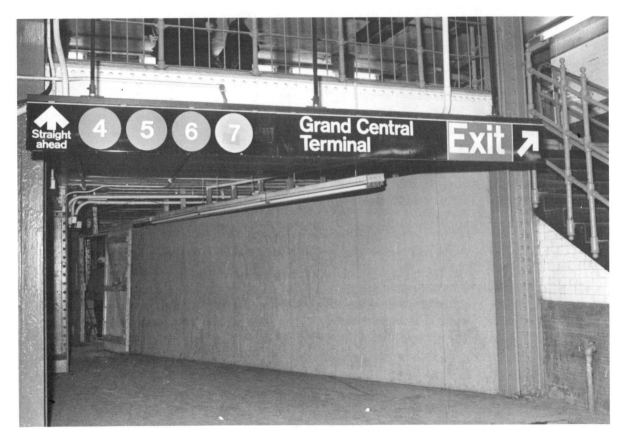

Isolated or empty passageways are among the areas to be avoided by deaf-blind travelers who are alone.

necessary. Although many deaf-blind persons desire to travel independently in spite of risks, there will be times when independent travel will have to be forfeited for safety's sake.

With appropriate communication skills and methods, a finely developed use of the remaining senses, alternative and supplemental mobility techniques, and a good measure of self-confidence, deaf-blind persons can be the independent travelers they want to be. Helen Keller, who never traveled independently herself but who was always on the arm of Anne Sullivan or Polly Thomson, was overwhelmed on the occasion of her 80th birthday when deaf-blind persons from all over the country came to the Industrial Home for the Blind in New York for the celebration. These people flew in by plane; took subways, trains, or buses to the event; or walked. Having achieved so much in her life, but never the skill of independent mobility, Miss Keller exclaimed at the time, ''At last I have seen deaf-blind people free.'' Despite the constantly changing and complex systems of mass transit today, the majority of deaf-blind persons enjoy an increasing amount of freedom of independent mobility.

References

Cote, J. (1987). Tactile Speech Indicator. *National Center News* (Helen Keller National Center), p. 33.

Fisk, S. (1986). Constant-contact technique with a modified tip: A new alternative for long cane mobility. *Journal of Visual Impairment & Blindness,* **80**(10), 999-1000.

Harrity, R., & Martin, R.G. (1962). The three lives of Helen Keller. New York: Doubleday.

Olson, R. (1986). SpecialNet. Federal Bulletin Board.

Wynne, Sr., B. (1982). *Population served at HKNC.* New York: Helen Keller National Center.

Wynne, Sr., B. (1980). *The power of touch: Communication and education.* New York: Helen Keller National Center.

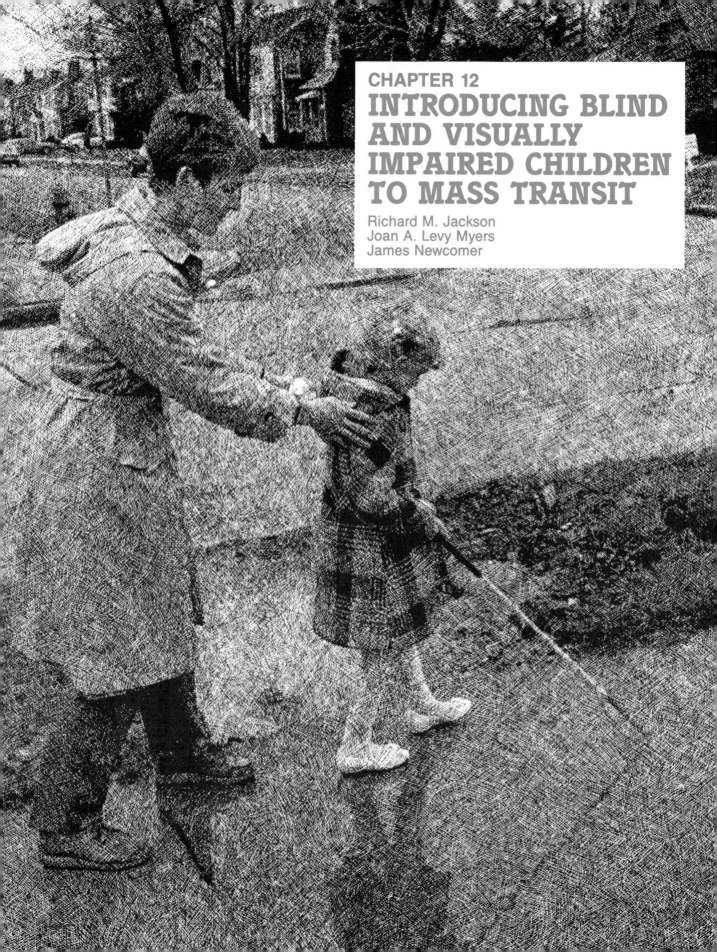

CHAPTER 12
INTRODUCING BLIND AND VISUALLY IMPAIRED CHILDREN TO MASS TRANSIT

Richard M. Jackson
Joan A. Levy Myers
James Newcomer

Orientation and mobility (O&M) specialists do not always agree about when to begin instruction in orientation to mass transit for blind and visually impaired children. In general, mass transit is dealt with later rather than sooner, but there is a growing awareness that at least an introduction to mass transit should be made early on. With more O&M specialists serving preschool and multidisabled children than ever before (although there are some areas in this country where there is still no O&M instruction), the introduction to mass transit for these youngsters can be a logical extension of the teaching curriculum. Although it is agreed that children must master many concepts and skills before they can be expected to travel independently, they can, at an early age, develop the confidence and desire to use mass transit when they are ready.

General Considerations

In general, a sound goal is to prepare children to be able to use mass transit for independent travel by the end of high school. At that point, it is typically expected that each student will have attained the necessary concepts and mobility skills to attend college, get a job, or live independently in the community.

Certainly, students must be given the opportunity to discover that public transportation can contribute enormously to their independence. It is not surprising that many blind and visually impaired people relocate to urban areas in their adult lives where they can have access to mass transit for the purpose of getting to and from jobs, availing themselves of community resources, and enriching their social, recreational, and cultural lives.

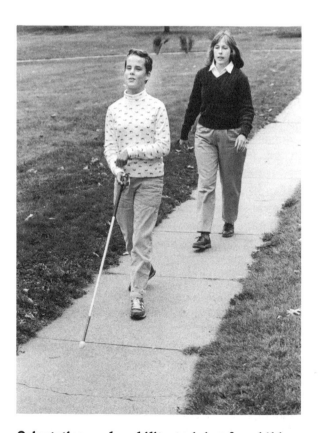

Orientation and mobility training for children should include particular skills required in mass transit travel.

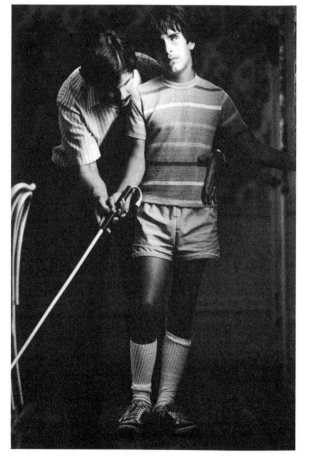

It is true that these activities require other skills in addition to O&M skills. College requires academic competence, employment requires vocational competence, and independent living in the community requires mastery of daily living skills. But competencies such as these may never be put into practice unless particular attention is paid to the O&M skills required to utilize the various modes of mass transportation. The aim of early educational programming in this area is to build the confidence, knowledge, and skill that eventually enable young persons to plan and negotiate a variety of routes incorporating all modes of travel.

At an early age, children become aware of buses, trolleys, trains, commuter rails, and, in some areas, rapid rail systems. They also discover that the automobile is the predominant and preferred mode of transportation in our culture. It is useful to consider a stage-linked approach to the teaching of mass transit travel skills to children. These stages would include awareness, exploration, discovery, utility, and mastery. Making sure that children become aware of mass transportation and its relevance to their lives requires careful planning and coordination of the traditional O&M curriculum with the regular education program and developmentally appropriate travel tasks. It also mandates a team approach—a team, for instance, that includes an itinerant teacher who has had experience in O&M or is served by an O&M specialist, the regular classroom teacher, a physical therapist, an occupational therapist, and the family.

Family Involvement
Teachers who work with blind and visually impaired students in suburbs or rural areas know the importance of involving students' families and helping them overcome their fears. Many family members often experience culture shock when they go to a nearby city; it can be difficult to encourage them to take their children on trains and subways, much less to let them travel independently.

Some families who are already fearful about allowing their children to travel alone express even greater reluctance when they contemplate mass transit. They may fear their children interacting with strangers, getting lost, or falling off a train platform. Such concerns are amplified all the more by the news media through stories of muggings, platform accidents, and random violence. These stories provoke and help sustain negative attitudes that can be directly or indirectly conveyed to the child. In the same way, the attitudes of siblings, peers, teachers, and others involved with the child can affect confidence and the desire to travel independently. Therefore, it is vitally important to maintain ongoing communication throughout a program with parents and others who play a critical role in the child's development. The child must have constant encouragement, direction, and support from all concerned.

If they can do so, family members need to travel with the child on the transit systems available in their own community. If they live in a rural area, they need to make the effort to obtain access to a transit system in an urban area at an early stage in the child's development.

Expansion of the School Curriculum
In the school curriculum, transportation is often a part of the unit on geography and modern life, and emphasis should be placed on making sure that children try to apply what they learn about transportation to their own personal lives. Otherwise, they may grow up feeling inferior if they learn only that the major mode of travel is the automobile and they know that driving a car is not an option for them. Even in casual conversation or simulated activity, students can be helped to develop positive attitudes about mass transit. Questions can stimulate them: If you want to go to the game, how would you get there? How much time would you need? If you want to take the train, where does the train take you?

Role-playing in simulation exercises also prepares students. In the same way that the teacher simulates street crossings and parallel traffic by using a sound box or another device, situations in mass transit can be imitated in the classroom.

In a flexible and creative curriculum, elementary school children should be getting some experience with buses, commuter trains, subways, and trollies.

Play materials can be introduced: every mode of public transportation has been represented in the toy industry for years. One can find automobiles, gas stations, airports, buses, trains, and train stations, and these toys, which can be manipulated or are three dimensional, often show what is critical and distinctive about the particular item. For example, toy buses show where people sit in rows, and toy trains show dining or baggage cars. Toys offer a variety of concepts that youngsters can explore and discover. Field trips can be used to reinforce this learning experience.

Field Trips

Although school scheduling may sometimes pose a problem, with some ingenuity and flexibility it is possible to set up field trips for different age groups. For example, an instructor can devote one day a month to travel in the city. Even if this is done once a year, if it is repeated for five or six years, it has cumulative value and deflects the anxiety a student might feel in the 10th or 11th grade when learning to travel to the city independently.

The type and amount of experience provided throughout a youngster's childhood play a crucial role in determining how much help will be needed later on. Many young children need experiences to understand concepts. If they get them at an early age, they are much more likely to use their skills as teenagers and put them to good use when they graduate. Students in residential schools that are in or close to a city have the advantage of the possibility of on-site mobility instruction. In some of the schools, passes to go off campus are given to capable high school students.

Plans for travel-related activities should be included in the Individualized Education Program (IEP) so that the objectives are clear. And they should be fun. In one city, the children visit the Library for the Blind, which supplies the Talking Books with which they are familiar, and meet the librarian. Special museums and historical sites can be worthwhile destinations as well.

Some instructors have been successful with group activities, and residential schools allow easy

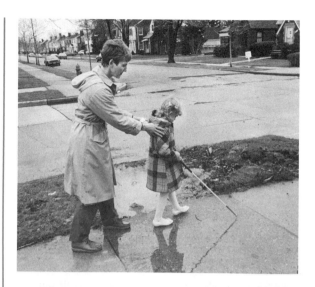

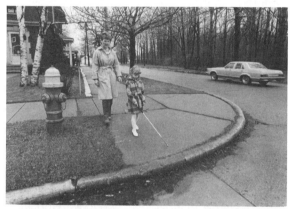

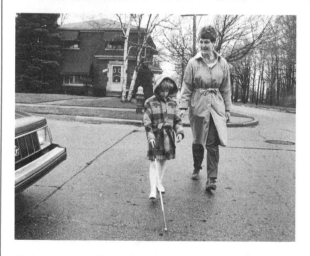

Even young children should be provided with experiences outdoors to prepare them for mass transit travel later in life.

access to such activities. Children as young as 4 have been taken on outings on transit buses or in school buses in areas where there is no public transportation. In the latter case, the teacher can make sure that the bus makes stops and that the children have distinct responsibilities for simulating a public transit bus ride. Dividing the duties allows those who have telescopic aids to identify the bus, others to ask the driver if they are on the right bus, others to tell the driver where they want to get off, others to sit next to the driver, and others to watch for landmarks. For motivation and incentive, there can be a picnic or lunch at a fast-food restaurant or a visit to a mall at the end of the ride.

To introduce children to mass transit, O&M specialists will have to analyze the locale, the situation, and the possibilities. They can do whatever is feasible, remain flexible, and be open to new opportunities. Children who are given the chance to explore and utilize their environment while being encouraged to develop highly integrated perceptual skills are most likely to achieve mastery in independent travel skills in later years.

Skills on the Secondary School Level

Procedures for teaching mass transit to blind and visually impaired students at the secondary school level are similar to those used when working with adults. However, blind and visually impaired children need additional help and practice in certain areas.

Cognitive, Social, and Emotional Skills

With the myriad of concepts and skills involved in the use of mass transit, it is important for the O&M specialist to determine how much actual planning and travel a child will ultimately be able to do independently. Previous experiences at home and school play a vital part in developing the child's skills and attitudes toward mass transit. However, cognitive, physical, and emotional functioning must be considered in determining ultimate level of independence. In addition, social behaviors, including manners, are generally learned at home. Situations may arise in which students behave in a manner inappropriate for the circumstances, such as when a student props his or her feet on the seat of a subway

train. Instances such as these require the instructor's intervention. Other similar situations may arise in which the instructor must help the student behave in a socially acceptable manner. This helps the student become less conspicuous in a variety of travel environments, which in turn fosters his or her confidence.

Map Reading Skills

Map reading should be a standard component of the O&M curriculum. The concepts involved in bus and train routes and general station layouts must be understood for route planning and maneuvering within stations. O&M specialists may debate about the amount of map reading skill necessary to facilitate efficient travel, but students should be given an opportunity to learn these skills so that travel is not limited to areas learned solely through repetition. Map reading skills increase a traveler's level of independence.

Telephone Skills

The acquisition of telephone skills helps blind and visually impaired students reach appropriate resources and obtain information for route planning. Many high school students lack both telephone etiquette and proper questioning techniques. In addition, they are not assertive, so that even if they learn the right questions to ask, they frequently are unable to obtain the necessary information.

Skills in using the telephone should be well developed either prior to or during instruction in bus travel. Routes should be planned by the student, not the instructor. When the instructor continually does the planning, the student will only be able to travel bus routes that have been planned by others. In general, it is difficult for students not only to plan a route, but also to apply their plan to a route incorporating the information.

By the time rapid rail travel is introduced, the student should only need guidance on efficient travel planning and selection of a preferred route. When trying to determine the direction from which to exit a particular train station, for instance, students learn that they should be specific when asking questions. For example, a student might ask, ''Do I exit toward the train's direction of travel?" or "Do I exit toward the front or back of the train?"

Skills for Soliciting Aid
Skill in soliciting help should be developed prior to instruction in mass transit. A student's previous experiences with soliciting aid will most likely have involved interaction with pedestrians. Additional instruction is necessary on how to ask bus drivers, street vendors, and other pedestrians appropriate questions for completing a route, as well as on how to assume the challenges of rapid rail travel. For example, it is important to familiarize students with the concept and usual location of a kiosk and the position of the microphone into which they must speak when talking to the clerk or attendant. Skills for soliciting aid when entering a train may also need to be developed. If a student desires to sit in designated handicapped seating areas or any other seat, he or she must find out if that seat is vacant. He or she may also have to ask questions to confirm the train's destination.

Skills for Obtaining Reduced Fares
The availability of reduced fares for disabled travelers and the procedures for obtaining them vary from city to city. It is important to inform blind and visually impaired students about reduced fares and to tell them that they have the option of paying the standard fare as well. If reduced fares are not available within stations, they must be purchased in advance at designated locations.

Skills for Obtaining Goods and Services
Blind and visually impaired students must have access to those places that may ultimately fill a variety of needs by providing goods and services. Mass transit can provide that access. After developing various skills, students can plan and negotiate routes to a number of places. It may be the first time that they will exit train stations and orient themselves once outside the station to an unfamiliar area. This phase of an instruction program is generally exciting and challenging. All previously taught concepts and skills must be well integrated into the students' planning and travel.

Even if students have achieved a high level of competence, they may still be apprehensive. During initial lessons, they should be observed while planning routes to make certain they obtain the necessary information for exiting from the correct side of the station and negotiating their route. The importance of soliciting aid when needed in an unfamiliar station environment, as well as confirming one's location outdoors, should be reinforced.

Students have an excellent chance of developing independent travel skills when these six areas for special consideration are integrated into an O&M training program for teaching mass transit travel. Adapting the program to meet their individual needs and levels of functioning, involving family and other people important in their lives, and instilling confidence will give blind and visually impaired children the freedom to travel in the future independently and confidently in many travel environments.

GLOSSARY

Auditory skills. The ability to interpret information about one's environment through the use of the sense of hearing.

Bioptics. Special telescopic lenses, mounted on conventional ophthalmic prescription eyeglasses, used for seeing distant objects in detail.

Clues. Any sound, odor, or sensation of temperature or tactile or visual stimulus that affects the senses and can readily be used in determining one's position or a line of direction.

Electric collector shoes. Devices attached to a train, which slide along the electrified third rail to transmit electricity from the rail to the train motors.

German measles. See **rubella.**

Landmark. Any familiar object, sound, odor, temperature, or tactual clue that is easily recognized and that has a known location in the environment.

Light rail. A form of transit, generally in cities and metropolitan areas, that uses street trackage and often has its private right-of-way.

Line of travel. The course along which a person is moving.

Localizing skills. The ability to orient oneself to the environment through the use of the sense of hearing.

Lower-arm and forearm technique. An orientation and mobility technique used to locate and provide protection from objects at waist level.

Mowat Sensor. A secondary electronic travel aid that can be used by dog guide and long cane travelers to locate bus-stop signs, benches, doorways, other landmarks, and pedestrians.

Rapid transit. An aboveground or underground passenger transportation system in urban areas that has its own right-of-way.

Retinitis pigmentosa. A chronic, progressive disease characterized by night blindness in the early stages, atrophy and pigment changes in the retina, constriction of the visual field, and eventual blindness.

Rubella. An infectious viral disease that is milder than typical measles but is damaging to the fetus when occurring early in pregnancy. Also known as German measles.

Search pattern. A systematic approach to locating or determining the position of an object or landmark.

Self-familiarizing technique. The ability to acquaint oneself with a new environment in a systematic fashion.

Shorelining. An orientation and mobility technique in which a blind person detects the border or edge of any walkway with a cane.

Signage. The form and style of signs used in mass transit systems to communicate way-finding information or directions on how to use the system.

Squaring off. The act of aligning and positioning one's body in relation to an object for the purpose of getting a line of direction perpendicular to the object and establishing a definite position in the environment.

Tactile warning tiles. Tiles that can be affixed to or embedded in the ground surface of a mass transit environment. The tiles are designed to be detectable underfoot and with a cane and are typically used to warn of danger, such as at the edge of a subway platform.

Telescopic aids. Devices used for seeing or magnifying distant objects.

Third rail. A metal rail through which electric current is led to the motors of any electrically powered rail vehicle.

Touch technique. The method of walking with a cane that has been developed for use by blind persons. In it, wrist revolution moves the cane's tip in a sweeping motion, causing it to contact the ground at a point just parallel to the outside of each shoulder. During walking, correct rhythmic manipulation times each sweep of the cane so that the cane and the heel of the foot on the opposite side of the body contact the walking surface in unison.

Variations of the touch technique for increasing drop-off detection include the **touch-and-slide technique,** in which the cane is allowed to slide a few inches along the surface after contact; the **touch-and-drag technique,** in which alternate cane sweeps are dragged across the surface; and the **constant-contact technique,** in which the sweeping cane is dragged across the surface without being lifted off the surface at all.

Trailing. The act of using the fingers or a cane to follow a surface for any or all of the following reasons: to determine one's position in space, to locate a specific objective, or determine a parallel line of travel.

Upper-arm and forearm technique. An orientation and mobility technique used to detect and provide protection from objects that may be encountered by the upper region of the body.

Usher's syndrome. Pigmentary degeneration of the retina associated with deafness.

Vision-reduction goggles. Goggles that simulate reduced visual acuity and restricted visual field.

RESOURCES

Organizations

Blindness

American Council of the Blind
1010 Vermont Avenue, N.W.
Suite 1100
Washington, DC 20005
(202) 393-3666
Promotes effective participation of blind people in all aspects of society and acts as a national information clearinghouse.

American Foundation for the Blind
15 West 16th Street
New York, NY 10011
(212) 620-2000; (800) 232-5463 (Hotline)
Provides direct and technical assistance services to blind and visually impaired persons and their families, professionals in specialized agencies for blind persons, community agencies, organizations, schools, and corporations.

Regional Centers

Mid-Atlantic Regional Center
1615 M Street, N.W.
Suite 250
Washington, DC 20036
(202) 457-1487
Serves Delaware, District of Columbia, Kentucky, Maryland, Ohio, Pennsylvania, Virginia, and West Virginia.

Midwest Regional Center
20 N. Wacker Drive
Suite 1938
Chicago, IL 60606
(312) 269-0095
Serves Illinois, Indiana, Iowa, Michigan, Minnesota, Missouri, and Wisconsin.

Northeast Regional Center
15 West 16th Street
New York, NY 10011
(212) 620-2032
Serves Connecticut, Maine, Massachusetts, New Hampshire, New Jersey, New York, Rhode Island, and Vermont.

Southeast Regional Center
100 Peachtree Street
Suite 1016
Atlanta, GA 30303
(404) 525-2303
Serves Alabama, Arkansas, Florida, Georgia, Louisiana, Mississippi, North Carolina, Puerto Rico, South Carolina, Tennessee, and the Virgin Islands.

Southwest Regional Center
260 Treadway Plaza
Exchange Park
Dallas, TX 75235
(214) 352-7222
Serves Colorado, Kansas, Montana, Nebraska, New Mexico, North Dakota, Oklahoma, South Dakota, Texas, and Wyoming.

Western Regional Center
111 Pine Street
Suite 725
San Francisco, CA 94111
(415) 392-4845
Serves Alaska, Arizona, California, Guam, Hawaii, Idaho, Nevada, Oregon, Utah, and Washington.

Association for Education and Rehabilitation of the Blind and Visually Impaired
206 North Washington Street
Alexandria, VA 22314
(703) 548-1884

Promotes all phases of education and work for blind and visually impaired persons of all ages. Operates a job exchange and reference information center. Certifies rehabilitation teachers, orientation and mobility (O&M) specialists, and classroom teachers.

Canadian National Institute for the Blind
1931 Bayview Avenue
Toronto, Ontario M4G 4C8
Canada
(416) 486-2636
Fosters the integration of blind and visually impaired persons into the mainstream of Canadian life and promotes prevention of blindness programs.

Canadian Rehabilitation Council for the Disabled
45 Sheppard Avenue East
Suite 801
Willowdale, Ontario M2N 5W9
Canada
(416) 862-0340
Acts as the principal national advocacy, coordinator, and resource center for organizations serving Canadians with disabilities.

Christoffel-Blindenmission
Nibelungenstrasse 124
D-6140 Bensheim 4
Federal Republic of Germany
06251-1310
Works with all aspects of blindness in more than 60 countries, with emphasis on the prevention of blindness and the treatment of eye diseases. Provides substantial support to education and rehabilitation services for blind persons.

Council for Exceptional Children
1920 Association Drive
Reston, VA 22091
(703) 620-3660
Champions the rights of exceptional individuals to full educational opportunities, career development, and equal employment opportunities.

Council of U.S. Dog Guide Schools
c/o Martin Yablonski, President
Guiding Eyes for the Blind
611 Granite Springs Road
Yorktown Heights, NY 10598
(914) 245-4024
Provides a forum for the exchange of information about successful operating practices employed by 10 member dog guide schools.

Helen Keller International
15 West 16th Street
New York, NY 10011
(212) 807-5800
Assists governments and voluntary agencies in developing countries in establishing and integrating services to prevent or cure eye diseases and blindness into their national health and welfare systems and in rehabilitating and educating blind and visually impaired persons.

Helen Keller National Center for
Deaf-Blind Youths and Adults
111 Middle Neck Road
Sands Point, NY 11050
(516) 944-8900
Provides technical assistance to facilitate transition of deaf-blind youths from education to community-based adult services through its Technical Assistance Center.

International Council for Education
of the Visually Handicapped
c/o Christoffel-Blindenmission and
Royal Commonwealth Society for the Blind
Southeast Asian Pacific Regional Office
4 Taman Jesselton
10450 Penang
Malaysia
Promotes the education of visually impaired people throughout the world and represents the interests of visually impaired children and those who teach them.

National Council of State Agencies for the Blind
206 N. Washington Street
Suite 320
Alexandria, VA 22314
(703) 548-1885
Promotes communication and coordination among agencies involved in preventing blindness and offering services to severely visually impaired individuals.

National Federation of the Blind
1800 Johnson Street
Baltimore, MD 21230
(301) 659-9314
Seeks the complete equality and integration of blind individuals into society. Monitors all legislation affecting blind people, evaluates present programs for blind persons, and assists in promoting needed services.

National Industries for the Blind
524 Hamburg Turnpike
Wayne, NJ 07470
(201) 595-9200
Provides technical, engineering, and administrative support to its associated industries to improve and increase job opportunities for blind Americans.

Office for Civil Rights
U.S. Department of Health and Human Services
330 Independence Avenue, S.W.
Washington, DC 20201
(212) 245-6403
Administers and enforces laws prohibiting discrimination on the basis of sex, race, color, religion, national origin, age, or disability in access to health care and social services receiving federal funds from the department.

President's Committee on
Employment of People with Disabilities
1111 20th Street, N.W.
Washington, DC 20210
(202) 653-5044

Seeks to eliminate physical and psychological barriers for disabled people through education and information programs; promotes education, training, rehabilitation, and employment opportunities for people with disabilities.

Royal National Institute for the Blind
222 Great Portland Street
London, W1N 6AA
United Kingdom
388 1266
Works for the welfare of all blind people in the United Kingdom.

World Blind Union
58 Avenue Bosquet
75007 Paris
France
45-55-67-54
Serves as coordinating agency for representatives of national associations of the blind and agencies serving blind people. Provides an international forum for the exchange of knowledge and experience in the field of blindness.

Transportation

American Institute of Architects
Department of Design
1735 New York Avenue, N.W.
Washington, DC 20006
(202) 626-7300
Strives to advance standards of architectural education, training, and practice.

American National Standards Institute
1430 Broadway
New York, NY 10018
(212) 354-3300
Acts as a national clearinghouse and coordinating body for trade associations, technical societies, professional groups, and consumer organizations regarding voluntary standards.

American Public Transportation Association
1201 New York Avenue, N.W.
Washington, DC 20005
(202) 898-4000
Seeks to represent the urban transit industry on an international scale, to provide safe, efficient, and economical transit services, and to improve those services to meet national energy, environmental, and financial concerns. Provides a medium for exchange of ideas and experiences; promotes research and investigation.

Architectural and Transportation Barriers Compliance Board
U.S. Department of Health and Human Services
South Building, Room 1004
330 C Street, S.W.
Washington, DC 20201
(202) 245-1591
Enforces standards that require certain federally funded buildings and facilities to be accessible to physically disabled persons.

Canadian Urban Transit Association
55 York Street
Suite 1105
Toronto, Ontario M5J 1R7
Canada
(416) 365-9800
Represents transit operators, suppliers, consultants, and government agencies to gather and distribute technical and operational transit information; provides a forum for transit-related issues; encourages transit research and development.

Institute of Transportation Engineers
525 School Street, S.W.
Suite 410
Washington, DC 20024-2729
(202) 554-8050
Represents transportation professionals from all over the world and conducts research, seminars, and training sessions; provides professional and technical information on transportation standards and recommended practices.

International Mass Transit Association
1190 National Press Building
Washington, DC 20045
(202) 662-7171
Strives to improve the public image of mass transport; promote the development, improvement, and expansion of mass transport; and encourage the financing of transport systems.

National Research Council
Institute for Research and Construction
Associate Committee on the National Building Code
Ottawa, Ontario K1A 0R6
Canada
(613) 993-9960
Represents building officials, producers and manufacturers, and construction professionals in the transit industry throughout Canada.

National Transportation Safety Board
Safety Programs
800 Independence Avenue, S.W.
Washington, DC 20594
(202) 382-6600
Promotes traffic safety through independent investigations of accidents and other safety problems. Makes recommendations for safety improvements.

Project ACTION (Accessible Community Transportation In Our Nation)
1001 Connecticut Avenue, N.W.
Suite 435
Washington, DC 20036
(202) 659-2229
Seeks to improve access to mass transportation services for people with disabilities through the development, demonstration, and dissemination of a cooperative model program. Administered by the National Easter Seal Society.

Royal Institute of British Architects
66 Portland Place
London W1
United Kingdom
580 5533

Represents British architects dedicated to the advancement of civil architecture.

Transportation Research Board
2101 Constitution Avenue, N.W.
Washington, DC 20418
A unit of the National Research Council that devotes attention to research in transportation systems planning and administration and in the design, construction, maintenance, and operation of transportation facilities. Holds an annual conference on transportation issues.

Union internationale des transports publics
(International Union of Public Transports)
Avenue de L'Uruguay 19
B-1050 Bruxelles
Belgium
2 6733325
Studies all problems connected with the private transport industry and suggests solutions with a view toward promoting the progress of private transport.

Urban Mass Transportation Administration
U.S. Department of Transportation
400 Seventh Street, S.W.
Washington, DC 20590
(202) 366-4040
Is responsible for the development of improved mass transportation facilities, equipment, techniques, and methods and assists state and local governments in financing mass transportation systems.

Orientation & Mobility Preparation Programs

Belgium

I.R.S.A.
Chaussu de Waterloo, 1504

1180 Bruxelles
Belgium
2-374-9090, Ext. 255

Koninklijk Institute Spermalie
Snaggaardstraat 9
B-8000 Brugge
Belgium
050-34-03-41

Federal Republic of Germany

Ausbildungsstatte fur Rehabilitationslehrer
fur Blinde und Sehbehinderte
Am Schlag 8
D-3550 Marburg 1
Federal Republic of Germany
(06421) 606-173, 606-174

Deutsche Blindenstudienanstalt's
(German Institute for the Blind)
Postfach 1160
D-3550 Marburg
Federal Republic of Germany
(06421) 606-773

Institute for Rehabilitation and
Integration of the Sight Impaired
Sierichstrasse 56
D-2000 Hamburg 60
Federal Republic of Germany
(0) 40/2700422

Padagogische Hochschule
6900 Heidelberg
Federal Republic of Germany
(06221) 477-410; 477-400

Ghana

National Mobility Centre
Accra, Ghana 227101

Israel

Migdal Or (American Israeli Lighthouse)
Rehabilitation Teachers Division
Kiriat Haim, Israel

Japan

Research Institute
National Rehabilitation Center for the Disabled
1, 4-chome, Namiki
Tokorozawa, Saitama 359
Japan
0429-95-3100

Netherlands

Dutch Association for the Blind
and Partially Sighted People
Utrecht
The Netherlands
040-443336

Stichting Revalidate van Blinde
en Slechtziende Volwassenen
(Rehabilitation Foundation for Blind
and Visually Handicapped Adults)
Waldeck Pyrmonstraat 31
7315 JH Apeldoorn
The Netherlands
055-21sllg

Theofaan Institut Voor Blinden en Slechtzienden
St. Elizabethstraat 4
5361 HK Grave
The Netherlands
08860-71003 (75919)

New Zealand

Massey University
Rehabilitation Studies Section
Department of Psychology

Palmerston North, New Zealand
69-099

Spain

La Laguna University
Didactic and Educational and
Behavior Research Department
La Laguna, Tenerife, Canary Islands
Spain
922/220303

ONCE (Organization Nacional de
Ciegos Espanoles)
Calle del Prado 24
28104 Madrid
Spain
1-429-96-42

United Kingdom

Royal National Institute for the Blind
Birmingham
United Kingdom
021-643-9912

United States

Arkansas

University of Arkansas at Little Rock
Department of Rehabilitation
Personnel Programs
33rd and University
Little Rock, AR 72204
(501) 569-3169

California

California State University at Los Angeles
Department of Special Education

5151 State University Drive
Los Angeles, CA 90032
(213) 224-3743

San Francisco State University
Department of Special Education
1600 Holloway Avenue
San Francisco, CA 94132
(415) 469-1080

Colorado

University of Northern Colorado
Division of Educational Studies
Greeley, CO 80639
(303) 351-1673

Florida

Florida State University
Visual Disabilities
College of Education
Tallahassee, FL 32306
(904) 644-4880, 644-4881, 644-4882

Illinois

Northern Illinois University
Department of Learning, Development,
and Special Education
DeKalb, IL 60115
(815) 753-8455

Massachusetts

Boston College/Graduate School
of Arts and Sciences
Department of Special Education
and Rehabilitation
McGuinn Hall B-29
Chestnut Hill, MA 02167
(617) 552-4181

Michigan

Michigan State University
Department of Counseling, Educational Psychology
336 Erickson Hall
East Lansing, MI 48824
(517) 355-1871

Western Michigan University
Department of Blind Rehabilitation
Kalamazoo, MI 49008
(616) 387-3455

Pennsylvania

University of Pittsburgh
School of Education
Department of Special Education
5M01 Forbes Quadrangle
Pittsburgh, PA 15260
(412) 624-1403

Tennessee

George Peabody College
Vanderbilt University
Department of Special Education
Box 328
Nashville, TN 37203
(615) 322-8160

Texas

Stephen F. Austin State University
SFA Station, Box 13019
Nacogdoches, TX 75962
(713) 569-2906

Texas Tech University
College of Education
Box 4560
Lubbock, TX 79409
(806) 742-2320; 742-2345

Sources of Equipment and Materials

Audible-Traffic Pedestrian Signal Devices and Braille Blocks

Aldridge Traffic Systems
6 Queen Street
Mitcham, Melbourne
Australia 3132

Coeval Products
99 Constitution Street
Leith, Edinburgh
Scotland, EH6 7AE

Dansk Signal Industry
P.O. Box 510
DK-2650 Hvidovre
Denmark

Edwards Company
P.O. Box 1188
Farmingham, CT 06034
(203) 678-0410

Nagoya Electric Works Co. Ltd.
1-36 Yokobari-Oho
Nakagawa-Ku, Nagoya
Japan

Sumitomo Seimei
Okayama Building
1-1-1 Yanagicho
Okayama City, 700
Japan
81-862 23-1711; FAX 81-862 25-2508

Traconex
366 Martin Avenue
Santa Clara, CA 95050
(408) 727-0260

Bus Number Identifiers

Compact Travel Aids
P.O. Box 69707
Seattle, WA 98168

Compasses for the Blind

BIAB Electronic
Verkstadsvagen 57
S-714 00 Kopparberg
Sweden

Marshmallow Cane Tips

Wurzburger Mobility Aids
3960 Cottonwood Drive
Concord, CA 94519

Mobility Guiding Systems for the Blind

Ikeno Tsuken Corporation
2-13-9 Higashi 10Jo
Kitaku, Tokyo 114
Japan
81-3 913-6191

Plastic Letter Writing Guides

Independent Living Aids
11 Commercial Court
Plainview, NY 11803
(516) 752-8080

Tactile Maps

Gilligan Tactiles
34 Kilburn Road
W. Newton, MA 02165

University of Maryland
Department of Geography
Joseph Weidel, Chairman
College Park, MD 20742
(301) 454-2241

Baruch College, City University of New York
Computer Center for the Visually Impaired
New York, NY 10010
(212) 725-7644

Tactile Speech Indicator

Helen Keller National Center for
Deaf-Blind Youths and Adults
111 Middle Neck Road
Sands Point, NY 11050
(516) 944-8900 (Voice and TDD, telecommunication
device for the deaf)

Tellatouch

American Foundation for the Blind
15 West 16th Street
New York, NY 10011
(212) 620-2000; (800) 232-5463 (Hotline)

BIBLIOGRAPHY

The following list contains materials that readers may find helpful.

Accessibility assistance: A directory of consultants on environments for handicapped people. (1978). Washington, DC: National Center for a Barrier-Free Environment and Community Services Administration.

American Foundation for the Blind. (1988). *Directory of agencies for blind and visually impaired persons in the United States, 23rd edition.* New York: Author.

Bentzen, B.L. (1989). *Considerations in the design of tactile maps for use by visually impaired travelers on rail rapid transit* (Report # UMTA-MA 06-0140-89-7). Washington, DC: U.S. Department of Transportation, Urban Mass Transportation Administration.

Bentzen, B.L. (1989). *Enhanced transit telephone information systems to promote accessibility of transit to visually impaired travelers* (Report # UMTA-MA-06-0140-89-7). Washington, DC: U.S. Department of Transportation, Urban Mass Transportation Administration.

Bentzen, B.L. (1989). *Laboratory research concerning tactile warning tiles to promote safety in the vicinity of transit platform edges* (Report # UMTA-MA-06-0140-89-3). Washington, DC: U.S. Department of Transportation, Urban Mass Transportation Administration.

Bentzen, B.L. (1989). *Specifications for letters and numerals for touch reading* (Report # UMTA-MA-06-0140-89-9). Washington, DC: U.S. Department of Transportation, Urban Mass Transportation Administration.

Bentzen, B.L., Jackson, R.M., & Peck, A.F. (1981). *Information about visual impairment for architects and planners* (Report # UMTA-MA-0036-81-2). Vol. 2 of *Improving communications with the visually impaired in rail rapid transit systems.* Washington, DC: U.S. Department of Transportation, Urban Mass Transportation Administration.

Bentzen, B.L., Jackson, R.M., & Peck, A.F. (1981). *Selection of tokens and orientation of farecards by visually impaired users of rail rapid transit.* (Report UMTA-MA-0036-81-4). Vol. 4 of *Improving communications with the visually impaired in rail rapid transit systems.* Washington, DC: U.S. Department of Transportation, Urban Mass Transportation Administration.

Bentzen, B.L., Jackson, R.M., & Peck, A.F. (1981). *Solutions for problems of visually impaired users of rail rapid transit* (Report # UMTA-MA-0036-81-1). Vol. 1 of *Improving communications with the visually impaired in rail rapid transit systems.* Washington, DC: U.S. Department of Transportation, Urban Mass Transportation Administration.

Bentzen, B.L., Jackson, R.M., & Peck, A.F. (1981). *Techniques for improving communication with visually impaired users of rail rapid transit systems* (Report # UMTA-MA-0036-81-3). Vol. 3 of *Improving communications with the visually impaired in rail rapid transit systems.* Washington, DC: U.S. Department of Transportation, Urban Mass Transportation Administration.

Bentzen, B.L., & Peck, A.F. (1989). *In-transit research concerning tactile warnings to promote safety in the vicinity of transit platform edges* (Report # UMTA-MA-06-0140-89-4). Washington, DC: U.S. Department of Transportation, Urban Mass Transportation Administration.

Bentzen, B.L., & Peck, A.F. (1989). *Tactile warnings to promote safety in the vicinity of platform edges: Laboratory testing of pathfinder tiles vs. "corduroy"* (Report # UMTA-MA-06-0140-89-5). Washington, DC: U.S. Department of Transportation, Urban Mass Transportation Administration.

Braf-Per-Gunnar. (1974). *The physical environment and the visually impaired.* Translated by William Pardon. Bromma, Sweden: ICTA Information Centre.

The Canadian National Institute for the Blind. (1987). *Access needs of blind and visually impaired travellers in transportation terminals: A study and design guidelines.* Canada: Author.

Detectable tactile surface treatment for visually impaired persons: Background materials for workshop, January 18, 1984. New York: American Foundation for the Blind.

Duncan, J., Gish, C., Mulholland, M.E., & Townsend, A. (1977). *Environmental modifications for the visually impaired: A handbook.* New York: American Foundation for the Blind.

Gill, J.M. (1986). *International directory of agencies for the visually disabled.* Middlesex, UK: Research Unit for the Blind, Brunel University.

Goldman, C. (1987). *Disability rights guide.* Lincoln, NE: Media Publishing.

Ground and floor surface treatments/U.S. Architectural and Transportation Barriers Compliance Board. (1983). Washington, DC: U.S. Architectural and Transportation Barriers Compliance Board.

Hill, E.W. (1986). Orientation and mobility. In Geraldine T. Scholl (Ed.), *Foundations of education for blind and visually handicapped children and youth: Theory and practice.* New York: American Foundation for the Blind.

Hill, E.W., & Ponder, P. (1976). *Orientation and mobility techniques: A guide for the practitioner.* New York: American Foundation for the Blind.

Irwin, R.B. (1955). *As I saw it.* New York: American Foundation for the Blind.

Jackson, R.M., Peck, A.F., & Bentzen, B.L. (1983). Visually handicapped travelers in the rapid rail transit environment. *Journal of Visual Impairment & Blindness, 77*(10), 469-475.

Joffee, E. (1984). Visually impaired travelers: The suburban environment. *Journal of Visual Impairment & Blindness, 78*(10), 493.

Jose, R.T. (Ed.). (1984). *Understanding low vision.* New York: American Foundation for the Blind.

Katzmann, R.A. (1986). *Institutional disability: The saga of transportation policy for the disabled.* Washington, DC: The Brookings Institution.

Kidwell, A.M., & Greer, P.S. (1973). *Sites, perception, and the nonverbal experience. Designing and manufacturing mobility maps.* New York: American Foundation for the Blind.

Kirchner, C. (Ed.). (1989). *Data on blindness and visual impairment in the U.S.: A resource manual on social demographic characteristics, education, employment and income, and service delivery, 2nd edition.* New York: American Foundation for the Blind.

Koestler, F. (1976). *The unseen minority: A social history of blindness in the United States.* New York: David McKay.

Lederman, S.J., & Kinch, D.H. (1979). Texture in tactile maps and graphics for the visually handicapped. *Journal of Visual Impairment & Blindness, 73*(6), 217-227.

Long Cane News. New York : American Foundation for the Blind.

Neustadt-Noy, N., Merin, S., & Schiff, Y. (1986). *Orientation and mobility of the visually impaired.* Jerusalem, Israel: Heiliger Publishing.

Passini, R., Dupré, A., & Langois, C. (1986). Spatial mobility for the visually handicapped active person: A descriptive study. *Journal of Visual Impairment & Blindness, 80*(8), 904-907.

Peck, A.F. (1989). *Considerations in the design of an auditory beacon for use in rail rapid transit* (Report # UMTA-MA-06-014089-2). Washington, DC: U.S. Department of Transportation, Urban Mass Transportation Administration.

Peck, A.F. (1989). *Enhancing access to rail rapid transit via an auditory pathway* (Report # UMTA-MA-06-0140-89-8). Washington, DC: U.S. Department of Transportation, Urban Mass Transportation Administration.

Peck, A.F., & Bentzen, B.L. (1987). *Tactile warnings to promote safety in the vicinity of transit platform edges* (Report # UMTA-MA-06-0120-87-1). Washington, DC: U.S. Department of Transportation, Urban Mass Transportation Administration.

Peck, A.F., & Bentzen, B.L. (1989). *Validation of techniques improving communication with the visually impaired in rail rapid transit* (Report # UMTA-MA-06-0140-89-1). Washington, DC: U.S. Department of Transportation, Urban Mass Transportation Administration.

Schenkman, B.N. (1986). The effect of receiver beamwidth on the detection time of a message from Talking Signs, an auditory orientation aid for the blind. *International Journal of Rehabilitation Research, 9*, 239-246.

Templer, J., Lewis, D., & Sanford, J. (1983). *Ground and floor surface treatments.* Washington, DC: U.S. Architectural and Transportation Barriers Compliance Board.

U.S. Architectural and Transportation Barriers Compliance Board. (1977). *Resource guide to literature on barrier-free environments with selected annotations.* Washington, DC: Author.

U.S. Architectural and Transportation Barriers Compliance Board. (1980). *A multidisciplinary assessment of the state of the art of signage for blind and low-vision persons: Final Report.* Washington, DC: Author.

U.S. Architectural and Transportation Barriers Compliance Board. (1982). Minimum guidelines and requirements for accessible design. *Federal Register, 47*(150), 33862-33893.

Uslan, M.M., Hill, E.W., & Peck A.F. (1989). *The profession of orientation and mobility in the 1980s: The AFB competency study.* New York: American Foundation for the Blind.

Uslan, M.M., & Schreibman, K. (1980). Drop-off detection in the touch technique. *Journal of Visual Impairment & Blindness, 74*(5), 179-182.

Uslan, M.M., Waddell, B.L., & Peck, A.F. (1988). Audible traffic signals: How useful are they? *ITE Journal*, 37-43.

Welsh, R.L., & Blasch, B. (Eds.). (1980). *Foundations of orientation and mobility.* New York: American Foundation for the Blind.

Wiedel, J.W., & Groves, P. (1969). *Tactual mapping: design, reproduction, reading, and interpretation* (Final Report RD-2557-S 1969). Washington, DC: Department of Health, Education, and Welfare.

Yeadon, A. (Editor and Compiler). (1988). *International Low Vision Directory.* Philadelphia: Pennsylvania College of Optometry.

ABOUT THE AUTHORS

Billie Louise Bentzen is research associate, Department of Psychology, Boston College, Chestnut Hill, Massachusetts.

Sam C.S. Chen is international program development manager, International Department, Telesensory Corporation, Mountain View, California.

Kathryn Chew is an orientation and mobility specialist and vision resource teacher, Edmonton Public School Board, Edmonton, Alberta, Canada.

Anne L. Corn is professor, Department of Special Education, and coordinator, Programs for the Visually Handicapped, University of Texas at Austin.

Donald J. Dzinski is director, Safety and Program Development, American Public Transit Association, Washington, DC.

Edwin Eames is adjunct professor, Department of Sociology, California State University at Fresno.

Toni Gardiner Eames is adjunct assistant professor, Department of Sociology, California State University at Fresno.

Ann Frye is director, Disability Unit, Department of Transport, London, England.

Toni Provost-Hatlen is an orientation and mobility specialist, Living Skills Center for the Visually Handicapped, San Pablo, California.

Samuel S. Hines is an orientation and mobility specialist, Virginia Department for the Visually Handicapped, Richmond, Virginia.

Richard M. Jackson is director, Division of Special Education and Rehabilitation, and associate professor and director, Projects in Visually Handicapped Studies, Boston College, Chestnut Hill, Massachusetts.

Robert O. LaDuke is associate professor, Department of Blind Rehabilitation, Western Michigan University, Kalamazoo.

Steven J. LaGrow is senior lecturer in rehabilitation studies, Department of Psychology, Massey University, Palmerston North, New Zealand.

Chester Lubecki is an orientation and mobility specialist and low vision consultant, Elwyn Institute, Elwyn, Pennsylvania.

Dave Manzer is coordinator, Special Education, Visually Impaired, Ministry of Education, Delta, British Columbia, Canada.

Mary M. Michaud is supervisor, Orientation and Mobility and Low Vision Department, Helen Keller National Center for Deaf-Blind Youths and Adults, Sands Point, New York.

Takuma Murakami is an orientation and mobility specialist, Tokyo Metropolitan Rehabilitation Center for the Physically and Mentally Handicapped, Tokyo, Japan.

Linda Alexander Myers is an orientation and mobility specialist, Living Skills Center for the Visually Handicapped, San Pablo, California. She is currently chairperson of the International Environmental Modifications/Architectural Barrier Removal Committee for the Association for Education and Rehabilitation of the Blind and Visually Impaired, Division 9.

Joan A. Levy Myers is an orientation and mobility specialist in Alexandria, Virginia. She is the chairperson of the Washington Orientation and Mobility Association, Washington, DC.

David J. Mueller is a special education teacher, Roanoke County Schools, Virginia. He was an orientation and mobility specialist, Dekalb County Schools, Georgia, at the time of writing.

James Newcomer is director, Special Education, Quakertown Community School District, Quakertown, Pennsylvania.

Clementine Newkirk is on-call service coordinator, Elderly and Handicapped Lift Bus Service, Washington Metropolitan Area Transit Authority, Washington, DC.

Alec F. Peck is associate professor, Department of Special Education and Rehabilitation, and senior research associate, Center for the Study of Testing, Evaluation, and Educational Policy, Boston College, Chestnut Hill, Massachusetts. He is co-author of *The Profession of Orientation and Mobility in the 1980s*, and has written extensively on the topic of visually impaired travelers in rapid rail environments, and has received several research grants in the past decade from the U.S. Department of Transportation.

Gloria Sanborn is the owner of Compact Travel Aids in Seattle, Washington, which distributes bus identifier kits. She is a member of the Visually Impaired/Deaf-Blind Task Force of the Seattle Metro Transit.

Osamu Shimizu is director, Konan Rehabilitation Center, Saitama, Japan.

Arlene Stern is a writer and editorial consultant in the field of human services. Formerly director of publications of the Child Welfare League, New York, New York, she has worked in both the for-profit and non-profit sectors. Her memberships have included the American Society for Association Executives and the Society for Scholarly Publishing.

Edward B. Stone is a teacher of visually impaired students and an orientation and mobility specialist, Gwinnett County Schools, Georgia.

Mark M. Uslan is manager, Technical Evaluation Services, National Technology Center, American Foundation for the Blind and was, at the time of writing, national consultant in orientation and mobility, American Foundation for the Blind. He is co-author of *The Profession of Orientation and Mobility in the 1980s*, and has conducted extensive research on orientation and mobility technology for blind and visually impaired people. He is a member of the steering committee of Project ACTION (Accessible Community Transportation in Our Nation), which seeks to improve access to mass transportation services for people with disabilities.

Charles H. Wacker, Jr. is research consultant, Foundation for the Junior Blind, Los Angeles, California.

Ralph S. Weule is department manager, Safety and Investigations, Bay Area Rapid Transit, San Francisco, California.

William R. Wiener is president-elect, Association for Education and Rehabilitation of the Blind and Visually Impaired, and chairperson, Department of Blind Rehabilitation, Western Michigan University, Kalamazoo. He is co-author of *Travel in Adverse Weather Conditions* and has written on the development of orientation and mobility as a profession and various aspects of mobility training.

INDEX

Walking, 133–134
Warning strip. *See* Tactile warning strips
Washington Metropolitan Area Transit Authority (WMATA), 45, 47, 49, 68
Washington Orientation and Mobility Association (WOMA), 45–47
Western Michigan University, 29, 130
Weston-Super-Mare, 96

What Do You Do When You Meet a Blind Person (American Foundation for the Blind, 1971), 99
Wheelchair accessibility, 59, 60
Writing, 145

Yamanote Line (Tokyo), 113
Yes, Yes-No System, 145

Photo credits

American Foundation for the Blind (AFB), pp. 15, 148; Bay Area Rapid Transit (BART), p. 53; Oraien Catledge, pp. 26, 33, 104, 107, 108, 110; Sam Chen, pp. 56, 115; Chicago Transit Authority, 3; Department of Transport, London, 103; Sally DiMartini, 134; Foundation for the Junior Blind, pp. 116, 117, 118, 121; French Government Tourist Office, p. 36, 85; Generalsekretariat SBB, cover, p. 34; Dolores Hanley, pp. 18, 93; Bradford Herzog, p. 153; Japan National Tourist Organization, cover, pp. 36, 55, 112; Living Skills Center for the Visually Handicapped, pp. 86, 88; Barbara Loudis, cover, pp. 4, 7, 8, 10, 12, 14, 16, 20, 21, 22, 27, 28, 29, 36, 63, 150; Russ Marshall, pp. 152, 155; Metropolitan Atlanta Rapid Transit Authority (MARTA), pp. 31, 39; Mary Michaud, pp. 136, 141, 144, 146, 148; Carol Morton, p. 153; T. Murakami and O. Shimizu, pp. 56, 113, 114; Joan Levy Myers, p. 130; New Mexico School for the Blind, p. 9; Singapore MRT Ltd., p. 58; TASS from Sovfoto, cover, pp. 36, 128, 132; Washington Metropolitan Area Transit Authority (WMATA), pp. 38, 44, 46, 47, 49, 50, 51; Wisconsin School for the Visually Handicapped, p. 13, 127.

It is the policy of the American Foundation for the Blind to use in the first printing of its books acid-free paper that meets the ANSI Z39.48 Standard. The infinity symbol that appears above indicates that the paper in this printing meets that standard.